Speech therapy:

a clinical companion

Speech therapy:
a clinical companion

NOTES ON CLINICAL PRACTICE
FOR STUDENTS

Jennifer Warner,
Betty Byers Brown and
Elspeth McCartney

Manchester University Press

©1984 Jennifer Warner, Betty Byers Brown
and Elspeth McCartney
First published 1984, reprinted 1988 by
Manchester University Press
Oxford Road, Manchester M13 9PL

Distributed exclusively in one USA and Canada by
St. Martin's Press, Inc., 175 Fifth Avenue,
New York 10010, USA

British Library Cataloguing in publication data
Warner, Jennifer
  Speech therapy
  1. Speech therapy
  I. Title   II. Byers Browns, Betty
  III. McCartney, Elspeth
  616.85'506   RC423
  ISBN 0—7190—0993—6

Library of Congress Cataloguing in Publication data
Warner, Jennifer
  Speech therapy
  Bibliography: p.
  1. Speech therapy for children. I. Byers Brown,
Betty. II. McCartney, Elspeth. III. Title [DNLM:
1. Speech therapy — In infancy and childhood. WM 475
W282s]
RJ496.S7W33 1983   618.92'855   83—18788
ISBN 0—7190—0993—6

Printed in Hong Kong
by Wing King Tong Co. Ltd.

Contents

Foreword

I am pleased to be asked to write a foreword for this book because the authors have managed to produce a substantial volume of work which is designed to be a practical guide to the practice of speech therapy with children. The book is essentially designed to give the therapist a detailed description of the techniques found to be most effective in the practice of their profession. The readers will be impressed with the detailed way in which the book is written so that every contingency usually encountered is explained and practical solutions offered.

Each chapter is written in such a way that clear guidelines are given so that the student entering this profession will have a textbook on which to base her practice when facing speech and language disorders, from the common ones to those encountered less frequently.

Whilst the book is written in a style which is designed to be of practical guidance the authors have managed very skilfully to point the reader in the direction of the literature as it affects the topic under discussion and where possible they have outlined the principles behind the practice.

January 1983   *Professor I.G. Taylor*

Introduction to the text

The profession of speech therapy in Great Britain has never taken kindly to the construction of stereotyped programmes of treatment. It perceives therapy to be a creative process in which procedures are used with considerable selectivity. Any idea that students should be trained by 'cookbook' techniques is repugnant to clinician and teacher alike. We associate ourselves with this view and have no wish to limit the approaches and techniques of any creative clinician. Nor do we wish to usurp the role of the clinical tutor whose responsibility it is to prepare the student for clinical practice and oversee her progress towards clinical competence.

The purpose of this Clinical Companion is to support students as they make their first venture into clinical work by offering guidance in a form which is easily available for reference, particularly at times of doubt or emergency. The structure of most courses of study is based upon formal teaching in all subjects contributing to the theory of communication disorders. Early observation of children developing normally and abnormally is also a feature of most courses. The syllabus then moves on to the specialised conditions of speech pathology and these are accompanied by clinical tutorials and clinical practicum.

However well integrated and well planned the course of study there is obvious difficulty in ensuring that students will be prepared for all aspects of clinical experience. It is usual for students to start their clinical work with young children and they swiftly find that a real child is so much more than a clinical example. This is why we have confined our first Clinical Companion to the child population. We have concentrated upon the more commonly presented problems of language and are aware of the many omissions in our text, particularly those of prosody, phonation and fluency. These topics are receiving attention in the research literature and we are likely to be given more information in the future as the working of feedback and regulatory mechanisms are clarified.

In the broad field of child language, students are already hard put to absorb the many ideas recently generated. It is extremely difficult for them to compress these ideas into clinical procedures particularly when confronted with the human problems involved in case management. We offer this guide in the attempt to help them. We have also endeavoured to set down some of the procedures which the profession has found useful but which have not necessarily been recorded in the literature.

We hope that this text will go some way to assuage the anxieties of students who are academically well prepared but clinically inexperienced. The appeals made to us as clinical tutors prompt us to believe that it is necessary. Memories of our own early predicaments prompt us to hope that it will be helpful.

CHAPTER 1

General introduction: clinical setting and the student's clinical responsibilities

Speech therapists employed by the Health Authority may work in a variety of clinical settings and the student's clinical placement may be at one or more of the following:

Health centre or community clinic
Assessment centre or children's department of the local hospital
Day-care centre or nursery school
Specialised pre-school unit or specialised clinic
Special schools for the physically handicapped, mentally handicapped, hearing impaired, language handicapped
Language units attached to normal or special schools

You must make yourself acquainted with how the service is organised and how any individual unit is run.

The following general points should be considered:

Your placement will have been arranged by agreement between your tutor and the clinician in charge who will have received a brief outline of your training and experience. It is important to fit in with the general clinical procedures and you must consult the clinician on all matters pertaining to the management of patients. At certain times there may be a gap between the theoretical aspects of your training and the demands made in your clinic. If any problems arise discuss these as soon as possible with your clinician or your tutor.

Whenever possible you should notify the clinician if you are are going to be absent, preferably in time for alternative arrangements to be made for your patients. Make sure that you have the telephone number of the clinic and if necessary the telephone numbers of the other places of work where the clinician can be contacted in an emergency.

Be punctual. It is probably advisable to arrive fifteen to twenty minutes before the clinic starts in order to collect equipment, prepare the room or discuss arrangements with your therapist.

The therapist in charge of the service will be required to make returns to the authority and will be asked to keep records in the format prescribed. You must make sure that you have completed attendance records before leaving so that they can be submitted to the person responsible for making statistical returns.

Find out how day-to-day treatment is recorded. You will probably be asked:

to write clear notes on *each treatment session* – these should give sufficient information for the speech therapist to continue work in your absence but be concise enough to be read quickly

and

to write a summary of the treatment and progress for each patient at the end of each term/clinical placement/patient discharge.

Remember that your clinician will have her own responsibilities during the session. Try not to disturb her work with patients unless absolutely necessary. If toys, tests and equipment are stored in the therapist's room try to plan ahead and collect anything you may need in advance in order to avoid interruption.

Make sure that you put equipment back in the appropriate place and notify the therapist if any materials are accidentally damaged by yourself or a patient.

Your therapist will probably tell you who will be responsible for you if she is unexpectedly absent. If she has patients booked in and you cannot treat them yourself, see them briefly, explain the situation and tell them to come for their next appointment unless they are notified.

If you are invited to observe the therapist working with patients remember to avoid anything that will distract or disturb the patient. Avoid taking notes during the session unless permission has been given.

Your therapist will know that you are required to keep a casebook as part of your clinical training. Access to the patients' notes and records is at the discretion of the therapist and you should always ask for permission to read the notes and make a summary.

Your therapist will be asked to send a report on your clinical work and she may observe some of your sessions. You must remember that complete clinical competence is not expected of you but your therapist (or tutor) will be looking for:

your ability to establish a supportive working relationship with your patients and their relative(s)

the suitability of your treatment — your timing, flexibility, choice of materials and your responses to the patient's success or failure

your choice of assessment procedures, the deductions that you have made and your awareness of additional problems or difficulties

your ability to consider the theoretical implications of the problem but above all your growing insight into the development of your own clinical skills.

You should remember that both your therapist and clinical tutor are there to advise and guide you and welcome discussion, questions and your willingness to enter into critical appraisal of your work.

Check whether your therapist likes you to wear a white coat, whether formal or casual clothes are accepted and, if tea or coffee are provided, whether you are expected to pay for these.

Clinical resources will vary according to monies available and other local conditions. You should make yourself responsible for your own routine equipment and not rely on the materials available at a clinic. The following suggestions for *basic* equipment are made:

felt pens or crayons

pictures to screen different phonemes for production and discrimination

pictures of 'minimal pairs'

pictures for language stimulation

a bag of small mixed toys or objects to stimulate/test naming and comprehension in young children:

   car

   doll

   teddy

   ball

   cup

   spoon

   shoe

   horse or pig

   chair or bed

one piece of equipment such as a ring-stack/pegboard for conditioning attention control, listening, imitation of sounds or words

simple picture form board for naming/modelling action phrases or easy verbal comprehension

cards or paper/scissors/sellotape.

Sources of information, sending letters and writing reports

This section deals with the collection, collation and dissemination of information. It is divided into two parts:

1. Information sources
2. Requesting further information and writing reports

It is essential to remember that all information on a child and his family is confidential. Anonymity must be maintained when discussing the patient outside the clinic setting and the student's personal casebook records should not contain facts that could lead to the identification of the patient. Data on a patient are given at the discretion of the therapist in charge and/or other professionals involved in the care and management of that patient. The student must consult her clinician before writing for additional information and obtain the parents' permission before sending or requesting reports other than to or from the original referring authority.

Information sources

Information on a patient can be obtained from a variety of sources including the medical or clinical records, reports from other professionals, school reports and the individual case history taken by either the speech therapist or the student. Reports and personal data may not always be available at the time of the first appointment. This is often the case with the handicapped child who may have been seen by a number of specialists in a variety of clinics or hospitals over a considerable period of time.

The summary in Table 1 outlines the areas that may need to be considered when attempting to build a diagnostic profile or planning appropriate treatment or management. Parents or caregivers will provide relevant information during the initial interview and case history but additional, detailed data may have to be obtained from the original source.

The summary outlines eleven areas for data collection divided into three sections:

A. Routine information
Identifying and admininstrative data

B. Basic clinical information
Personal history
Speech and language development
Vision and hearing
Family history
Educational history

C. Additional information for specific disorders
Cranio-facial disorders including cleft palate
Development delay including mental handicap
Neurological impairment including cerebral palsy
Disorders of hearing and vision
Disorders of behaviour and mood

Table 1   Data collection

A. Routine information: required for clinical records/further appointments/obtaining and sending reports

Identifying and administrative data

Information	Sources
Name	
Age Date of birth	
Name and address of General Practitioner	
Source of referral	
Date of referral	
Address of: 　　　School 　　　Unit 　　　Assessment centre 　　　Nursery school 　　　Play group	Medical or clinical records Referral letter
Name of: 　　　Head teacher 　　　Class teacher 　　　Unit or remedial teacher 　　　Nursery or play group 　　　　supervisor	Confirmation by parents at initial interview
Name and address of other professionals involved: 　　　Medical consultant(s) 　　　Psychologist 　　　Physiotherapist 　　　Occupational therapist 　　　Health visitor 　　　Social worker	
Hospital or clinic number (if applicable)	
Date of initial interview with Speech therapist	

B. Basic clinical information: required for diagnosis/treatment and management

Personal history

Information	Sources
(a) Development history: vegetative functions/social development/mood and behaviour/motor abilities/ cognitive abilities	Medical or clinical notes Reports from relevant consultants: paediatrician/neurologist/surgeon/E.N.T. consultant/psychologist/G.P.
(b) Medical history: health/illness/ recurrent complaints/accidents/ operations/medication	Developmental checklists given to parents before initial interview
Investigations and assessments: date/place/professional concerned/ results	Parents' comments at interview
(c) Birth history: health of mother and child/pre-/peri-/post-natal factors	Student's own observations

Speech and language development

Information	Sources
Developmental history including previous speech therapy assessments and treatments	Parents' comments at interview
	Reports from speech therapist previously concerned with the child
Dual language or multi-language systems	School or nursery school report
	Student's own observations at initial interview

Vision and hearing

Information	Sources
Visual and/or audiological assessments: dates/place/tests used/results	Reports and audiogram from audiologist or E.N.T. consultant
	Reports from ophthalmologist
	Medical or clinical notes
	Parents' comments at interview

Family History

Information	Sources
Medical history	Parents' comments at interview
Details of parents and siblings	Reports from health visitor or social worker
Particulars of other household members	Report from G.P.
	Medical or clinical notes
Adult mainly responsible for care of the child	
Social/ethnic/environmental factors	
Particulars of housing	

Educational history

Information	Sources
Information on special school placement	Parents' comments at interview
	Reports from school or unit
Specific learning difficulties/subjects and achievements	Report from educational psychologist
Remedial teaching	
School refusal or truancy	
Parent satisfaction and involvement with school	

C. Additional information for specific disorders

Cranio-facial disorders including cleft palate

Information	Sources
Size, shape and relationship of cranio-facial structures/type of cleft/associated or additional skeletal abnormalities	Medical or clinical notes
	Reports from surgical team/dentist/orthodontist/oral surgeon/speech therapist/paediatrician
State of dentition and occlusion	
	Parents' comments at interview
Surgical intervention: date/place/type of primary or secondary surgery/tonsilectomy or adenoidectomy	
Additional intervention: prosthesis/dental or orthodontic treatment	
Measurements of velopharyngeal closure and air-flow dynamics: lateral cineradiography/videofluoroscopy/nasal endoscopy/nasal anemometry: assessments/results and conclusions	

Development delay including mental handicap

Information	*Sources*
Paediatric or neurological developmental history: physical and cognitive growth/abnormalities of sensory-motor systems/epilepsy/medication	Medical or clinical notes Reports from paediatrician/ paediatric neurologist/geneticist
Genetic or chromosomal history	Report from clinical or educational psychologist
Psychometric evaluation: date/place/ tests used/conclusions and recommendations	Reports from school or assessment centre
Educational placement and associated learning problems	Developmental checklists Parents' comments at interview

Neurological impairment including cerebral palsy

Information	*Sources*
Paediatric and neurological assessment: type of disorder/causal factors/nature of lesion/progressive or non-progressive/ upper motor neurone or lower motor neurone involvement/presence of spasticity/athetosis/ataxia/flaccidity	Medical or clinical notes Reports from paediatrician/ paediatric neurologist
Associated physical/sensory/cognitive disabilities	Reports and discussion with physiotherapist or occupational therapist
Level of reflex behaviour/vegetative functions/mobility/independence	Report from clinical or educational psychologist
Medication and intervention	Reports from school or assessment centre
Treatment by other professionals, e.g. physiotherapist/occupational therapist	Developmental checklists Parents' comments at interview
Psychometric evaluation: date/place/ tests used/conclusions and results	

Disorders of hearing and vision

Information	Sources
Audiological details: date(s)/place/ form of investigation – full assessment or screening test/tests used – distraction, co-operative, performance, free field or closed-circuit audiometry, impedance measurements/results/ recommendations	Medical or clinical notes Reports from E.N.T. consultant/audiologist/teacher of the deaf/health visitor/ophthalmologist Reports from school or assessment centre
Surgical or medical intervention: myringotomies/grommets/adenoidectomy or tonsilectomy/decongestants	Parents' comments at interview
Hearing aid(s): type/recommended settings	
Visual details: date(s)/place/form of investigation/type and degree of visual defect	
Surgery/intervention/glasses – type and when to be worn	

Disorders of behaviour and mood

Information	Sources
Details of behaviour: hyperactive/ apathetic/aggressive/destructive/ stereotype/obsessional/phobic/ritualistic/attention-seeking/temper tantrums	Medical or clinical notes Report from consultant child psychiatrist or clinical psychologist
Details of mood: anxiety/apprehension/ depression/withdrawal/mood swings	Report from social worker or health visitor
Somatic and vegetative disorders	Report from school
	Parents' comments at interview
Relationship and affections	Student's own observations at initial interview

Requesting further information from other sources and writing reports

In order to form a diagnostic opinion and advise on appropriate treatment and management the therapist or student requires as much information as possible on a child. Ideally, this information should be available at the time of the initial interview, case history or assessment. For a variety of reasons this may not be possible in practice and requests for additional information may have to be made following the child's first visit. The usual procedure is to write to the person or authority concerned.

Letter writing
The following points should be observed:

The recipient should be addressed by his or her professional title and name.

Letters should be clearly dated, signed, indicate the profession of the writer and student status.

Basic identifying information should appear as a heading at the start of the letter.

If your clinician wishes copies of the letter to be sent to others involved in the welfare of the child a list of their names and occupations should be included below your signature under the heading *Copies sent to*:

The letter should indicate whether the child is being seen for speech and language assessment, parent guidance, regular treatment or reassessment and explain succinctly the reason for requesting additional information or further investigation. Permission of the original referring authority should be obtained before the request is made.

If there is uncertainty about the name of the recipient every endeavour should be made to find this out before sending the letter. This can usually be done by telephoning

Figure 1. Basic format for professional letters

Reference number	Address of sender Telephone number Extension
	Date

Dear *Professor/Dr (physician or those*
   with doctorate degrees)
   Mr Ms (surgeon)/Mr Mrs Miss Ms
	Name

Re   Patients name
   Address
   Hospital number
   School address
   Source of referral
	Date of birth } *Essential*
	{
	{ *When*
	{ *applicable*

Yours sincerely,

Signature

Student Speech Therapist

Clinician's countersignature

Copies sent to:
Name   Profession

the hospital clinic, area health authority, educational authority or school.

Writing reports

The fundamental purpose of writing a report following speech and language evaluation or giving a resumé of treatment and management is to communicate relevant information clearly and succinctly. The following points should be considered:

The report should start with a heading *Speech therapy report*, should be dated and signed with the name and professional status of the writer.

The report should contain basic identifying data (name/ date of birth/address) and relevant administrative information (hospital number/school address/name and address of General Practitioner).

Statements should be simple and direct and the use of specific terminology kept to a minimum unless the recipient is familiar with the terms used.

Standardised or objective tests of speech and language should be referred to, in the first instance, by the full name followed by the abbreviated name or initials in brackets, for example, *Reynell Developmental Language Scales* (R.D.L.S.). The initials may then be used for subsequent references in the report to the test. Raw data from a test need not necessarily be included but mean scores, standard deviation scores and age levels should be clearly presented together with a brief description of the child's response to the test and the conclusions drawn from the test results.

Data obtained from systematic observations should be preceded by a description of the activity being observed, the time spent on the task and the level of spontaneity or adult direction. It is not always possible to make a definitive statement from observed behaviour and the report should indicate clearly that the comments and conclusions made, relate to the session(s) observed and may not be a complete description of the child's abilities or difficulties.

If specific information, for example the results of audiological assessment, is not available at the time of your own evaluation it is important to state this in the report so that the recipient is aware that your comments have been made in the absence of pertinent data.

A report is frequently presented in the form of a narrative statement. Subheadings may be used to help organise the information, but it is important to note that a report differs from a case history. The latter is a collection of data on a patient whereas a report should contain explanations, comments and conclusions as well as facts.

Try to distinguish fact from inference and state clearly whether an attitude is your own or that of another informant. Use a first-person reference to yourself to indicate when an opinion, evaluation or conclusion is yours rather than that of another professional or the parents.

A report on treatment and/or the progress made by a child should state which aspects of speech and language have been the main focus for intervention. Details of treatment techniques need not be included unless the recipient is also undertaking similar work with the child, for example, another speech therapist or the child's teacher. The report should state whether the treatment has been carried out by the student during a number of regular sessions or whether the main emphasis has been on the provision of a guidance programme for the parents or teacher. A progress report should include retest scores, if available, and a description of the child's present level of competence compared with his performance at the time of referral. Whenever possible some form of prognosis should be given. If progress has been un-satisfactory and a request for further investigation is being made the report should contain a short explanation and out-line the main reasons for supporting the request.

Avoid derogatory or critical comments about other pro-fessionals or the parents or care-givers. If some form of critical comment is essential for the well-being of the child the report should be factual and objective. Whenever possible the subject should be discussed with the person(s) concerned before the report is sent.

In the main section of the report refer to the child by name or personal pronoun and avoid frequent use of terms such as 'the patient' or 'the subject'.

Keep a report as short as possible. Use paragraphs to indicate a change of topic and in the final paragraph present a concise summary of the salient features, your conclusions and re-commendations.

Indicate clearly when you are presenting exact examples of the child's utterances. Do not use phonetic symbols if the recipient is unfamiliar with these. When quoting samples of the child's phonology include the target word as well as the example of the child's production.

Do not send reports without the permission of the therapist in charge and always ask for your report to be seen if you are in doubt or concerned about the content.

It may also be necessary to send detailed programmes for implementation by other people. These are considered further in Chapter 2 under parent counselling.

This chapter has been mainly concerned with administrative information. The assessment, treatment and management of patients is considered in the later chapters.

CHAPTER 2

Contact with parents or care-givers
Interviewing: taking a case history and counselling

Contact with the parents or care-givers of the speech-handicapped child is an integral part of patient management and an ability to interview and counsel with skill and empathy must be acquired. This will take time and practice.

When you have become familiar with the clinical setting and gained some experience, the therapist in charge may suggest that you interview the parents and take a case history or assume responsibility for counselling them on your treatment programme. You may feel some anxiety at first and question your ability to relate to and support the adults concerned. It is important to remember that most parents will readily accept you in your clinical role knowing that you are assisting the speech therapist.

This chapter covers aspects of the case history interview, review appointments and parent counselling. Table 2 illustrates the main occasions when contact is made between the adults responsible for the child and the therapist or student.

The demands made on you and the depth of your relationship with the parents will vary according to the reasons for the interview, the circumstances under which it is conducted and the personalities involved. Interviewing and counselling require flexibility, sensitivity, insight into the parents' reactions and your own feelings towards them and a knowledge of the extent and limitation of your professional role. You must be prepared to accommodate, to deal with a variety of responses and learn to reserve your judgement until you have met the parents on a number of occasions or talked to them for some time.

Your relationship with the parents or care-givers

You should consider the following points:

It is important to understand the influence of the parents' ethnic, social and religious backgrounds and to recognise that attitudes and principles may differ fundamentally from your own.

The exchange of information may be restricted and unintentional misunderstandings occur if the parents' command of English is limited. An interpreter or another member of the family may be needed at the interview but he or she should be someone the parents know and trust.

Parents' priorities may differ from your own and may not centre on the child's speech. They may be more concerned about other aspects of their child's development, behaviour or education. If you consider speech and language remediation to be a priority, give your reasons clearly and allow time for the parents to discuss the situation with either the therapist in charge or yourself.

Some parents may not appreciate at first that their child's delayed development of speech is related to a more general developmental delay or additional handicap. Comments on diagnosis, the child's behaviour or developmental levels should be reserved until you have some insight into their opinions, know how much they have already been told and gauged their readiness to accept new information.

The parents' previous experience with other professionals will influence their attitude towards you. Some will already have received sound information and advice, others may be confused by conflicting opinions or feel that they have not received adequate support in the past.

Whilst parents may lack your objectivity, they have the advantage of an intimate knowledge of their child on a day-to-day basis. You must learn to appreciate and make full use of their comments and to consider them together with your own observations.

You will also meet parents who have more experience of a specific handicap than you have yourself. Recognising and acknowledging their skill will help rather than hinder your relationship.

Parents have considerable demands made on their time. They may have other regular professional appointments, be involved in caring for younger children or older relatives or be at work. Fluctuating attendance or failure to continue a programme at home may not necessarily indicate a lack of concern or interest.

Very occasionally you will come into contact with parents whose attitude and behaviour towards their child causes you anxiety. If you are in any doubt about the relationship, discuss this with your therapist so that she can contact the appropriate person if necessary.

Finally, remember that although you are there to offer help and a professional service, not all parents will wish to take up this offer.

The case history interview

Purpose and form

The purpose of the case history and initial interview is twofold.

In order to gain some understanding of the child's difficulties and plan a future course of action or therapy, *the interviewer* needs time to gather information on the child and to verify and clarify facts already obtained from other sources. *The informants* need an opportunity to present the problem as they see it, to discuss their anxieties and priorities and to obtain answers to some of their questions.

Table 2 Contact between the adults responsible for a child and the speech therapist or student clinician

Purpose of contact	Nature of contact	Members of family involved	Professionals involved
Case history: Interview(s) to obtain data for assessment and the planning of future action or treatment	One occasion contact only e.g. special diagnostic clinic or assessment clinic	Adult* + child	Therapist + other professionals Student assisting or observing
	Initial contact at preliminary interview +	Adult* + child	Therapist + student or
	opportunity for extended contact on future visit(s)	Possibly adult* alone	student alone
Follow-up visits: Interview(s) for review and evaluating progress	Sporadic visits but family known to interviewer or infrequent visits and family new to the interviewer	Adult* + child / Adult* + child	Therapist + student or student alone
Parent guidance: Interview(s) for advice and guidance on maintaining ongoing treatment at home	Regular contact: Interviewer a familiar person	Adult* + child	Therapist + student or student alone
Special counselling: Interview(s) for help and counselling in an area of special expertise	One or two visits but family may be accompanied by another familiar professional who will give continued support	Adult* + child or adult* alone	Therapist or therapist + another professional Student observing
* Adult may be:	Both parents Mother or father alone Another member of the family Care-givers		

The interview should be considered as a dialogue between the adults concerned with the child and yourself. It should take the form of a directed conversation in which information is given, received and exchanged rather than a series of questions. When taking the case history you may initiate the topics and direct the discussion but the relationship between you and the parents should allow for freedom and spontaneity. In your role as a listener, a careful balance has to be maintained between genuine professional interest and concern and over-involvement. You should also remember that the case history interview is primarily a time for obtaining factual information and opinions and is not an occasion for altering or attempting to change attitudes.

Preparation for the interview

Setting the scene
Whenever possible the interview should be conducted in a quiet room free from disturbance and interruptions.

Important information, however, may sometimes be imparted casually in the waiting room or corridor. You may not be able to follow it up immediately but should make a note of it and return to the subject at a more appropriate time.

If you are meeting the parents for the first time the therapist in charge will probably introduce you. If not, make sure that they know your name and that you are assisting the speech therapist at the clinic.

Welcome them in a warm, relaxed manner and check that they are comfortable before beginning the interview.

Management of the room and the people involved
If another professional, for example a teacher or social worker, accompanies the family he or she may well take part in the interview. It is important that the parents know that they are the main focus of your interest and care has to be taken not to make them feel excluded from any part of the discussion. It may be better to invite the parents in on their own at the beginning

of the session and suggest that the other person joins later. However, some families know the accompanying person very well and may be reassured by his/her presence throughout the interview.

The arrangement of the room and seating needs some consideration. Much will depend on whether you are seeing the parents on their own or with their child. When the child is present care has to be taken not to expose him to discussion that might have a detrimental affect on him. If he is willing to play by himself or with an older sibling, place the adult chairs some distance from the child's table and move over to them when he is happily occupied and settled with some toys. Keep the interview short and concentrate on basic, factual information. If necessary the parents can be offered an opportunity to return on their own for an extended or more detailed discussion. Alternatively, you may suggest that they bring another member of the family, friend or neighbour on their next visit to care for the child for part of the session.

The slightly older child may be mature enough to tolerate separation from his family but anxiety or suspicion can be created by asking the child to wait in another room whilst you talk to his parents. It may be better to have him in the room with you and include him to a certain extent in the discussion. If he is happy to wait outside he should be reassured that he can come back into your room at any time and should be welcomed on his return.

When working with a teenager it is important to obtain his views and feelings and at least part of the interview should be conducted with him, possibly on his own.

Being informed

Before starting the interview try to be well prepared. Give yourself time to read any letters or reports on the child and his family. Note pertinent facts that might influence the direction of your enquiry or topics to be handled with care, for example, divorce, bereavement or aspects of the medical history.

Allowing time

When taking a case history it is advisable to allow for additional time and an extended session may have to be arranged. Interviewing cannot be rushed and a tight time schedule can create a feeling of tension which may be interpreted as disapproval or disinterest. Significant facts and comments are often presented towards the end of an interview when the parents are more relaxed and know you better.

Conducting an interview

Recording information and making notes

Many clinics provide a printed case history form as part of the standard clinical equipment. This should be used as a record document rather than a guide to the order in which questions are to be asked. You should ensure, however, that the relevant sections for essential clinical records and organisation are completed during the interview.

Always write down factual information such as dates and the names of the professionals and institutions concerned with the child, but whenever possible, lengthy note-taking should be kept to the minimum. With practice you will learn to rely increasingly on memory, supplemented by telegrammatic notes and signs and develop a technique for reminding yourself of the salient points and content of the interview.

Avoid writing down subjective, personal comments about the child and the family whilst the parents are present. These may be seen and cause anger or distress. Ideally the bulk of the writing should take place after the end of the interview when you have time to collate and organise the information and include considered opinions.

Using a tape recorder

The use of a tape recorder during an interview needs careful consideration. Most parents are happy to have an assessment or treatment session recorded but may be reluctant to have personal information put on tape. If you do decide to tape record the case history interview, the parents' permission should be obtained and you should explain that this is to allow you freedom to listen without making notes.

Explaining the purpose of the case history
Do not assume that the person interviewed understands the purpose of the interview or the reasons for some of the questions. Parents will expect to talk about their child's speech and language but may be unprepared for questions on general development and behaviour or the family history and circumstances.

At the onset of the interview talk to the parents about the case history. Explain briefly why you need detailed information on a range of topics and how this information will be used to help your assessment of their child.

Acknowledging information
If you have previously been given facts about a child and his family it may be helpful to acknowledge that you have received a letter or report from a specific person. This can be reassuring and act as a useful starting point for the discussion. However, acknowledging the receipt of information does not necessarily mean that you share the content with the parents. If they ask what another professional has said about their child suggest that they discuss it with the person concerned as you may not have received all the relevant facts.

How to begin
Start the interview by asking for simple factual information followed by a general question about the parents' opinion of the child's development or progress. This will provide an opportunity for you to evaluate the degree of insight attained by the parents and will help you set the level of the following discussion and questions.

How to proceed
As the interview progresses direct the discussion to specific

topics. One of the earliest should focus on the child's speech and language difficulties as parents will undoubtedly expect to discuss these with you and you will need their opinions in order to plan appropriate questions in other areas.

Many of the following topics will pursue causal factors. The extent to which you explore each one will be governed by the information you have already received, the parents' willingness and ability to provide the information and the circumstances of the interview.

During the course of the interview you should try to cover the areas described in the previous chapter.

Asking questions and ways of eliciting information
As you gain practice with interviewing you will develop your own approach and procedure. Consideration should be given to the various ways of encouraging discussion and obtaining facts.

In the non-directive approach, information is obtained by free dialogue and reflection. This is probably the best method for finding out about the parents' attitudes, opinions and feelings. Open questions often lead to this form of interchange.

The direct approach is used more frequently when specific or relatively predictable information is required. A series of direct questions can elicit appropriate, non-equivocal facts speedily leaving more time for the less predictable aspects of the case history.

A balance needs to be found between the two styles in order to obtain the maximum amount of information without disrupting or impeding the course of the interview unnecessarily.

Try to frame your questions clearly, ask them in a direct manner and listen to the answers carefully in order to pick up points for further clarification or expansion.

If you have to ask questions about personal problems be succinct, matter of fact and straightforward. Having asked the question wait for the reply without prompting.

Handling different responses and reactions
Whilst most parents will be clear historians, others may be very talkative and yet fail to provide relevant facts. Once you have allowed them to talk freely for a period of time you may have to find a way to interrupt the recital, be more assertive and redirect the discussion to appropriate areas.

Sometimes the information given by the parents may not seem relevant at first. Do not move on too rapidly as the most unexpected topic may reveal hidden anxieties or unanticipated problems and provide additional insight into the child's difficulties.

Inevitably you will meet some parents who become upset and distressed during the interview. Do not be too sympathetic as this may exacerbate their loss of control. Handle the situation either by expressing understanding and then presenting a new question on a less emotive topic or by giving the person time to gain composure by occupying yourself with another task for a short while.

You may occasionally meet parents who are hostile or aggressive and reluctant to take part in the interview. In this case, keep the case history short, concentrating on factual questions and focus your attention on the child as soon as possible. Once they have seen you working with and responding to their child they may be reassured and more willing to talk to you.

Answering the parents' questions and dealing with discrepancies
If the parents ask you questions try to answer them directly and honestly. When you do not know the answer either explain the reason, offer to find out for their next visit or refer them to an appropriate person.

When discrepancies occur between the parents' account and information from other sources, pursue the points tactfully and whenever possible check with the original source. During the interview contradictions and inconsistencies may occur. Do not enter into an argument but return to the point later in the discussion and try to gain clarification by approaching the subject unobtrusively and in a different manner.

Bringing the interview to a close

When you have obtained the information you need and feel you have covered the essential areas you should bring the interview to a close. End by asking the parents if they feel that the most important aspects have been covered and if they have any final questions. Explain any following procedures or appointments and make sure that they know who will be responsible for further decisions and recommendations.

Interviewing at review or follow-up appointments

A number of children and their families will return to the clinic for reassessment or review. Treatment may not have been advised at the time of the initial visit and the therapist may have recommended a follow-up appointment in order to evaluate spontaneous development or progress. Alternatively, regular treatment sessions may have been suspended for a period of weeks or months and a review appointment arranged in order to monitor progress and estimate whether the level of improvement has been maintained.

The attitude of the parents and the child in these circumstances will vary considerably. Some families will be very familiar with the clinical setting and the staff. Their relationship with the therapist will already have a sound foundation and they may have met you on previous visits. The interview is likely to be informal and relaxed and the parents will talk freely with the minimum of encouragement. Other families will have visited the clinic less frequently and may be meeting you for the first time. The relationship will be more formal and you may have to take a greater part in initiating and directing the discussion.

If you are meeting the parents for the first time it is important to reassure them that you are familiar with their child's previous history, development and treatment and before the interview you should study the clinical records carefully.

During the interview you should direct the discussion to a number of topics in order to obtain information on:

The parents' opinion on the progress made in speech and language development since their last visit and whether any new problems have occurred. Whenever possible, ask them to give specific examples of their child's speech to support their comments.

The degree of satisfaction or concern felt by the parents and their opinion on the need for therapy to be instigated or continued on a regular basis.

Changes that have occurred in the family, schooling, health and behaviour of the child that may have had a beneficial or detrimental effect on progress.

Specific advances that have been made in other areas of development and the effect that these have had on the child's speech.

Additional medical or educational assessments or retests of hearing and vision that have taken place in the intervening time.

Any additional help the child is receiving from other sources, for example, remedial teaching/peripatetic service for the hearing impaired/physiotherapy.

You may decide to reassess the child yourself before talking to the parents or following your initial discussion with them. The results of your assessment should be presented to them and the decision to instigate or continue regular treatment or discharge the child should be a joint one between the parents, the therapist in charge and yourself.

Counselling and guidance: helping parents supplement treatment at home

Children may attend clinics on a daily, weekly or infrequent basis depending on the nature and form of the treatment being undertaken, the individual circumstances of the family and the recommendations of the speech therapist. In any event, the parents or care-givers are concerned with the maintenance of treatment and the management of the child between visits. An essential part of most intervention programmes designed for young children is the counselling and advice given in order that supportive work can be continued in the child's home. Parents vary in their capacity and ability to work with their children but most will appreciate constructive help and many will become expert.

When you take over the treatment of a child the therapist may ask you to be responsible for planning and providing a parent programme and helping to implement this. In the final section of this chapter some general points are made about parent guidance but considerable flexibility is needed as no two families are the same.

Give positive help

If it is necessary to alter the attitude towards a child's behaviour or change the parents' responses or reactions to their child's speech, positive instructions and suggestions are more constructive than negative ones. Tell the parents what to do and how to do it as well as what they should avoid.

Observe the parent/child interaction before you give advice. Parents have their own skills and strengths and you should build on these. Radical changes in individual styles of interaction are difficult to achieve in the relatively short time you have with the family. Some adults are naturally more assertive and inclined to direct and control. Help them by showing how their energies can be used at an appropriate level for the child and when they should take a more passive role. Other adults adopt a more non-directive style. Encourage them to respond to their child's lead and show them how this can foster interaction and support and extend communication.

Give possible objectives

Set realistic goals for both the child and the parents and do not give too many instructions or suggestions at any one time. Find out what the parents are already doing and try to use this as your starting point.

Remember that the circumstances and atmosphere in the home may be very different from the more structured setting of the clinic. Ask the parents to suggest the best time and place to work with their child and show them how everyday activities can be incorporated into the programme if they are worried about setting aside a specific time.

Unless an absolutely consistent approach is needed suggest that older siblings or other members of the family can share the responsibility and undertake some of the work.

Give encouragement

If the parents are daunted by the prospect of working with their child and lack confidence in their ability to carry out suggestions give them time before providing a programme. Simply watching you work may be the most helpful form of instruction. They may try out some of your techniques at home and ask for further suggestions later, of their own accord.

Give demonstrations and written suggestions

Guidance is best given by combining three approaches.

(a) *Demonstration* – letting the parents watch you work with their child.
(b) *Discussion* – talking to them about what you have done and how it can be implemented at home.
(c) *A written programme* – giving them detailed instructions, reminders and further suggestions.

Ideally the parents should be given time to try out some of your suggestions during the session so that you can clarify any misunderstanding and they can ask questions as the need arises.

In certain circumstances you may not wish to have the parents in the room whilst you are working with their child. In this case you must allow sufficient time at the end of a session to explain any work you wish them to do between visits.

Demonstration and discussion

Do not worry if you make errors during a demonstration. A less than perfect session is often more useful as the parents can learn from your mistakes, particularly if these are discussed later.

Before inviting the parents to watch a session it may be beneficial to explain the aims and rationale for the chosen activities. It can also be helpful for you to suggest that they observe and note *specific aspects of your work*, for example one or more of the following:

Presentation and choice of materials: the need for one activity at a time: when to change activity to maintain interest and attention

Pace of work

Use and ways of prompting: physical/non-verbal/verbal

Timing of prompts: allowing the child sufficient time to respond before intervening/not leaving the child too long so that frustration or loss of attention occurs

Choice of rewards: those that are inbuilt into the activity/completion of the task/physical rewards/verbal responses/allowing the child to do something of his own choice on completion

Use of additional cues to supplement verbal instruction: gesture/cadence/the context of the situation itself

Using and accepting language at an appropriate level for the child

Ways of bringing about change of response from the child

Ways of increasing the complexity of the task

How to support the child and encourage him to continue a task

When to accept the child's attempt and when to demand more

How and when to 'correct' the child's utterances

You must remember that many of the points made above are implicit in your work and may not be obvious. The parents will need help to recognise them.

The written programme
Many parents express the need for written instructions to remind them of a session when they get home. If these are to be of use they must contain adequate detail and often take time to prepare, especially if you are uncertain beforehand how a child will respond. It is sometimes helpful to write the home programme after the session and send it to the parents by post after it has been agreed by the therapist in charge.

Keep the instructions short and simple but with sufficient information to support the parents if all does not go according to plan.

The following headings may help you when you are compiling more complex programmes:

General comments about the session and how the child responded. Give positive comments first

The aims of your suggested activities

General procedures for organisation and timing of the programme

A list of the activities and the materials that need to be available or prepared in advance

Specific procedures for each task and ways to respond to the child's anticipated reactions

How to cope and what to do if the child does not co-operate or fails to join in

How to extend the activity or invent new ones if the child learns quickly

Specific example of the vocabulary/grammatical structures/ sounds to be worked on

Suggested ways of keeping a record of progress

Additional counselling

Inevitably during your contact with parents your advice will be sought on the management of general behaviour or differing aspects of learning and development. You will have to rely on a combination of common sense and your knowledge of the learning processes and normal developmental sequences of young children.

You should consult your therapist if specific advice is requested on areas requiring either a specialised knowledge or information about local services and educational placement.

CHAPTER 3

Assessment and evaluation: general information

Although the speech therapist is primarily concerned with the assessment of spoken communication, her evaluation has to take into account medical and behavioural factors and the overall developmental competence of the child. Previous chapters have described the gathering of information from additional sources and emphasised the contribution of the parents or care-givers towards the appraisal of the problem.

The aim of this chapter is to summarise some of the assessment procedures that may be carried out by a speech therapist or by others concerned with the medical or educational well-being of the child. Information and data from these assessments contribute towards a diagnostic conclusion and act as a directive to the student clinician for selecting appropriate treatment or management. It should be remembered that assessment is an ongoing and continuous process and forms an integral part in any therapeutic relationship. Successful therapy is based on forming a treatment hypothesis from the initial assessment and subsequent careful monitoring and re-evaluation as each new treatment strategy is selected and introduced.

Assessment priorities

The starting point of any assessment is dependent on what is already known about a child and his problem. The speech therapist's *choice* of assessment procedures is governed by the child and his ability to interact and respond. The *interpretation* of the results and responses obtained will be influenced by information provided by others. As hearing impairment and mental handicap are the two major factors contributing towards delayed language acquisition certain information is essential to the speech therapist if realistic interpretations of language behaviour are to be made. The results of audiological evaluation are a priority in the assessment of the speech-impaired child. Until the child's hearing levels have been established, it is difficult to estimate the influence of other causal factors and how much they account for the speech and language delay. Psychological evaluation may also be essential in order to estimate the balance of the child's abilities. In certain circumstances this may not be part of the routine initial assessment. A psychological evaluation may be requested to support an opinion or confirm a speculative diagnosis. The same is true to a certain extent of detailed medical or neurological examinations. The speech therapist may suspect a condition from the speech assessment and ask for further investigations to verify the position. These interrelated aspects of assessment are illustrated in Figure 2.

Range of assessment procedures

Due to the complex nature of language and communication behaviour a number of aspects of the system have to be assessed. Developmental immaturities and a wide range of multiple handicaps exacerbate the problem still further. Factors influencing the range of speech and language assessment procedures and possible causal correlations are summarised in Figure 3.

Assessments should be seen as a process of detection based on a series of questions and logical steps.

The condition

What aspects of the child's speech and language must be evaluated in order to describe the problem?
Assessment choice: the linguistic dimensions of syntax, semantics, phonology and articulation and their function in production and comprehension.

Figure 2. Aspects of assessment: channels of access to information.

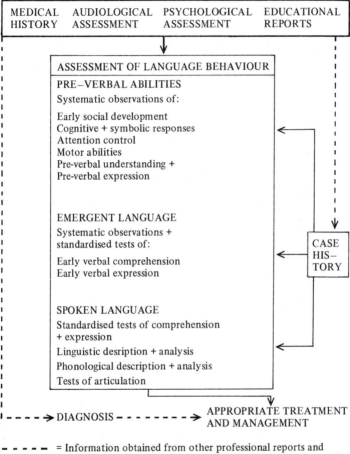

| MEDICAL HISTORY | AUDIOLOGICAL ASSESSMENT | PSYCHOLOGICAL ASSESSMENT | EDUCATIONAL REPORTS |

ASSESSMENT OF LANGUAGE BEHAVIOUR

PRE–VERBAL ABILITIES
Systematic observations of:

Early social development
Cognitive + symbolic responses
Attention control
Motor abilities
Pre-verbal understanding +
Pre-verbal expression

EMERGENT LANGUAGE
Systematic observations +
standardised tests of:

Early verbal comprehension
Early verbal expression

SPOKEN LANGUAGE
Standardised tests of comprehension
+ expression
Linguistic desription + analysis
Phonological description + analysis
Tests of articulation

CASE HIS–TORY

DIAGNOSIS

APPROPRIATE TREATMENT
AND MANAGEMENT

- - - - - = Information obtained from other professional reports and assessments

————— = Information that can be obtained directly by the student clinician

Figure 3. Assessment categories

ASSESSMENT PROCEDURES	THE PROBLEM	CAUSAL CORRELATES

Group I *Non-speaking children*

The child whose communication skills are extremely limited. There may be little attempt to interact by either verbal or non-verbal means. Vocalisations may occur but the extra linguistic cues of stress and prosody may be absent

or

The child who has failed to develop speech but attempts to interact by alternative means such as pointing, gesture and vocalisations accompanied by stress and prosody

Assessment by building up a developmental profile through systematic observations of the child's behaviour
A linguistic framework of description and standardisation tests may not be feasible

Causal correlates:
Early childhood autism
Severe mental retardation
Severe neuromotor impairment
Severe sensory loss
Specific developmental language disorder

Group II *Children who are attempting to use spoken language despite the limitations imposed by the speech handicap*

The child whose delayed language acquisition is part of a more general developmental delay

or

The child who presents with delayed language development but relatively normal development in other areas

Assessment by linguistic analysis of spontaneous and elicited speech + the use of standardised tests of speech and language together with complementary observational data

Causal correlates:
Moderate/mild mental retardation
Moderate/mild neuromotor impairment
Moderate/mild sensory loss
Specific speech and language delay

The method

What form(s) of assessment would be most appropriate for a specific child?
Assessment choice: norm-referenced and criterion-referenced tests; observational techniques; transcriptions and analysis of language sample.

Additional problems

What other abilities may need assessing if the child fails at an expected level?
Assessment choice: related processes that underpin language such as symbolic functioning; social competence and non-verbal interaction; attention control; auditory discrimination skills; motor ability.

Additional information

What additional information is needed in order to interpret the assessment or language behaviour?
Assessment choice: results of audiological, psychological and medical assessments; parental information.

Conclusions and inferences

What conclusions can be drawn from the overall assessments?
Choice: the presence of a significant problem; the nature of that problem and possible causal factors; appropriate treatment or management; the absence of a problem and the need to review or reassess.

Methods of assessment

A careful and thorough assessment is necessary to determine the existence of a problem and it is an essential prerequisite for effective therapy. A variety of assessment procedures may be undertaken with any one child. These may include observational techniques, the use of recognised tests and the recording of the child's utterances followed by detailed transcription and analysis.

Some tests are designed to indicate a child's attainment relative to that of children of a similar age. These *norm-referenced tests* provide standardised scores and compare an individual child's achievements with the performance of others within a relevant population. *Criterion-referenced tests* assess the child's mastery of a given task and are used when the clinician wants to know what the child can do rather than how he compares with others. Their purpose is to establish the individual child's progress towards a stated criterion and to inform the therapist where to start intervention. *Observational techniques* are frequently used to supplement and/or confirm the measures derived from the use of recognised tests. Judgements are based on systematic observations of the child's behaviour in a structured or free context and further inferences are drawn from whether that behaviour can be modified by adult intervention or interaction. For these techniques to be successful it is necessary to obtain a representative sample of the child's behaviour and performance and to devise ways of recording the observations.

Remember that you can also add to the details you obtain for yourself in the clinic by asking the mother or care-giver to provide information on the child's abilities and behaviour. It is helpful to give the adults concerned some direction on what to look for and record. Developmental scales, charts and checklists form a valuable guide. These are described in various texts or are published individually.

Example

> *P.I.P. Developmental Charts*, Jeffree and McConkey (1976)
> Age 0–5 years

This assessment covers five developmental areas, divided into subsections with a hierarchy of skills drawn up in each defined area. The charts provide a way of recording the individual child's development and progress. Age equivalents are also given.

The mother may also be used to elicit a language sample in the clinic if the child is reluctant to communicate with you initially, or you feel that you have not obtained a satisfactory representation of the child's output. Ask the mother if she would be willing to play and talk with her child and agree to you tape recording the conversation. Explain that this will give you the additional sample of her child's speech you need for later *transcription and analysis*.

It is unlikely that any one assessment procedure will supply all the information required and you should aim to master various assessment techniques and become familiar with the tests that are available. You will have been introduced to a range of tests and assessment procedures during the course of your academic studies and in your clinical practice you will gain experience in the administration of these tests and the interpretation of your test results.

Assessing the child's linguistic output

The most common features which are assessed in this area are vocabulary, syntax, content and phonology. It may also be necessary to assess the suprasegmental features of intonation and stress and more recently assessment procedures have also included the evaluation of the child's use of language and social interaction.

Examples of tests and assessment procedures

The Reynell Developmental Language Scales (RDLS), Reynell (1977) (revised) Expressive Scale: Age 6 months to 6 years

This scale is divided into three sections:

Scale 1 covers early vocal behaviour, the use of definite words and word combinations. These are elicited by the assesser or accredited by parents' comments.

Scale 2 assesses vocabulary through object and picture naming and by verbal means alone.

Scale 3 assess content and ideas through describing pictures.

The expressive scale is used in conjunction with the scale for comprehension (see page 000).

A Language Assessment, Remediation and Screening Procedure (LARSP), Crystal, Fletcher and Garman (1981) Age: 9 months to 4½+ years

This assessment procedure concentrates on the analysis of the child's grammatical structures. A sample of the child's language is obtained and a transcription is made which also includes information on prosody, stress and context. The transcription is then analysed for detailed grammatical information and a linguistic profile is build up for the child concerned.

The Edinburgh Articulation Test (EAT), Antony, Boyle, Ingram and McIsaac (1971) Age: 3–6 years

This test provides both quantitative and qualitative information on the child's articulation and developing phonology. The raw score obtained can be converted into a standard score and an articulation age. The authors also suggest that a standard score of eighty-five or less indicates the need for further detailed investigation.

The Goldman-Fristoe Test of Articulation (GFTA), Goldman-Fristoe (1972) Age: 6–16+ years

This test provides a systematic way of assessing articulation for single words and conversational speech. The manual gives qualitative interpretations and diagnostic interpretations.

Assessing the child's verbal comprehension

The most common features which are assessed in this area are the child's ability to understand basic vocabulary, grammar and meaning and interpret increasingly complex instructions.

If the child demonstrates difficulties with verbal comprehension it may also be necessary to test auditory discrimination skills or evaluate general symbolic abilities and the child's knowledge of objects, events and their relationship.

Examples of tests and assessment procedures

The Reynell Developmental Language Scales (RDLS), Reynell (op cit) Verbal Comprehension Scales A and B

Scale A tests the child's ability to understand single words by identifying objects or pictures and the ability to relate two objects or perform more complex activities in response to verbal instructions.

Scale B can be used with physically handicapped children who have poor motor control or with the shy or withdrawn child.

The test can also be modified for use with the hearing impaired. Standard scores can be obtained for both the Expressive Scale and the Verbal Comprehension Scale and age levels can be computed.

The English Picture Vocabulary Test (EPVT), Brimer and Dunn (1973) Age: 3–18+ years

This test assesses the child's comprehension of spoken vocabulary and provides standard scores, percentile scores and a vocabulary age.

The Test For Auditory Comprehension of Language (TACL), Carrow (1973) Age: 3–7 years

This test measures auditory comprehension of language structure and the relationship between grammar and meaning. Raw scores can be converted to age scores and percentile scores.

Derbyshire Language Scheme, Knowles and Masidlover (1982)

This scheme provides objective measures for evaluating early symbolic abilities, verbal comprehension and expression. The detailed manual also gives programmes to facilitate appropriate intervention.

Symbolic Play Test, Lowe and Costello (1977) Age: 1–3 years

This test evaluates levels of representational play (without language). Scoring is based on objective observations of the child's behaviour and raw scores can be converted to age levels.

You will find several other tests and assessment schemes in the clinics. If you come across an unfamiliar test discuss it with your clinician and ask to look at the manual, test materials and score sheets. You might find it helpful to keep a list of the tests available and add to it as new ones are presented to you. This provides a useful list as a reference and may help you in the selection of appropriate tests for an individual child.

The timing of formal assessment

This needs some consideration and will vary from child to child. If the child is apprehensive or reluctant to commit himself until he is familiar with the tester and the surroundings, it may be better to delay the administration of standardised tests until the latter part of the first session or postpone the testing until the second or third visit. The child should always be given time to settle and gain confidence and have every opportunity to demonstrate his highest and most successful levels of ability as well as his areas of difficulty.

The use of standardised tests: practical considerations

Read the manual carefully to become familiar with the procedures for the administration of the test. Note particularly:

what materials are needed and whether these are provided with the test or whether you must supply them yourself;

how the materials/pictures/word lists should be presented;

how the instructions should be given and how often (or not) they may be repeated;

whether there is a time factor for the completion of any part of the test;

when and why the test should be curtailed or ended;

how the responses should be notated, collated and recorded;

how the raw score(s) are converted to the standard score(s);

how often the test can be repeated and what period of time must elapse between test and retest.

You should also:

Check the test materials and forms before starting the test. Remember that the materials may have been part of the standardisation procedure and replacement of a missing piece with an alternative may invalidate the test.

If the child is allowed to help, for example turning the pages of the book or placing out objects, it may alter the speed of the test or increase the problem of controlling the situation. Make sure that comments to guide or control the child do not include test vocabulary.

Keep your verbal responses neutral. Avoid falling into the habit of rewarding success by comments such as 'Good' whilst responding to failure by silence. Take care not to give additional clues and if the placement of the materials is not stipulated in the manual remember to use a random system.

For tests that include a section on expressive skills check whether the test allows for models to be given and how imitated responses are scored.

If the parents or care-givers are present you may wish to give an outline of the purpose of the test and explain that the child is not necessarily expected to succeed in all sections. Tell them that there are rules for the administration of the test and remind them not to join in or help by giving extra information.

Oral examination: investigation of the size, shape and relationship of the cranio-facial structures and the function of the speech mechanisms

---

This should be a routine part of the assessment undertaken by a speech therapist. In certain circumstances a more detailed appraisal of the cranio-facial structures is needed and the child may already be under the care of the medical or dental services.

At the present time there are few norms or objective measures that can be applied to the oral examination of young children and judgements are largely subjective. In older children the speech therapist has to take into account successful compensatory measures adopted by the child that may counter-balance the structural abnormalities.

Equipment:

small pen torch
tongue depressors
cotton wool or paper tissue
small mirror

Procedure:

try to carry out the oral examination when the child is relaxed and confident in you;

explain to the child that you are going to look at his mouth and reassure him that it will not hurt;

if you are going to touch any part of the oral cavity with a tongue depressor or your finger tell him what you intend to do;

reassure a young child by letting him look in your mouth first or pretend to examine his mother, doll or teddy;

remember that good views of the oral cavity can be obtained if the child is laughing/yawning − be an opportunist and examine whenever a chance occurs spontaneously;

be relaxed yourself and initiate the examination without fuss or lengthy introductions;

if the child refuses, move on to another task and try again later.

Table 3 Oral examination

Examine	Note
General size, shape and relationship of the cranium and facial features	Marked abnormalities of the cranium/orbits/external ear/proportion of skull size to face
Size, shape and relationship of upper and lower jaws, dental arches and occlusion	Whether the teeth are well aligned and the upper and lower arches are in correct anteroposterior and lateral relationship
	Whether the lower jaw is too far back in relationship to the upper dental arch and skull (Angle's Class II)
	Whether the lower jaw is too far forward in relationship to the upper

Examine	*Note*
	dental arches and skull (Angle's Class III)
	Whether there is an openbite/close-bite/crossbite
Size, shape and position of teeth	Misalignment or displacement of teeth occurring with a normal relationship of the upper and lower dental arches (Angle's Class I)
	Missing/rotated/supernumerary/mis-aligned/displaced/hypoplatic teeth
Size and shape of maxilla, external nose and nostrils	Whether the maxilla is underdeveloped and the cheek bones look flat
	Whether the nose is excessively small/large/misshapen/deflected
	Whether the nostrils are small/flared/distorted/asymmetrical
	Whether there is a patent nasal airway or whether mouth breathing is habitual
Hard palate	The height/depth/width
	The presence, place, number and size of any fistulae
	The presence of any scarring or abnormal shadows or notches
Soft palate	The length/size/shape
	The presence of any scarring/a bified uvula/notching at the junction of the hard and soft palate
And velopharyngeal closure	The mobility of the soft palate and degree of elevation for 'ah'
	Whether the movements are sluggish or sharp

Examine	*Note*
	Whether a gag reflex can be elicited if palate appears immobile for speech
	Whether a small mirror 'mists' for test words requiring oral emission of air only (crude measure of nasal escape)
Lips	Posture at rest and during swallowing
	The presence of spasticity/flaccidity/tremor/choreo-athetoid movements
	The ability to maintain lip closure and resist attempts to open the lips
	Speed of voluntary lip movement
	Ability to spread/round the lips
	Symmetry of smiling and other movements
Tongue	General posture and position at rest
	Presence of spasticity/flaccidity/tremor/choreo-athetoid movements
	Abnormal posture or position: tongue thrust/retracted posture/curled or bunched posture
	Movements for chewing and swallowing
	Speed/range/strength/accuracy of movements
	Ability to move tongue without jaw movements/degree of compensatory jaw movement
Sensitivity	Ability to detect light touch (cotton wood, paper tissue or tongue depressor) and indicate the area of the oral cavity stimulated

Examine	Note
	Oversensitivity to touch leading to exaggerated responses
	Lack of sensitivity to touch
Reflex responses	Presence of expected reflex behaviour, e.g. gag reflex
	Presence of persistent immature reflex responses e.g. sucking reflex/biting reflex
Habit factors	Persistent use of dummy
	Thumb or finger sucking
	Biting of lips/tongue/inside cheeks
	Teeth grinding
Movements for speech	Imitation of vowels and consonants
	Imitation of non-linguistic syllables
	Imitation of linguistic utterances of increasing length e.g. 'but' 'butter' 'buttercup'
	'but' 'butter' 'butterfly' 'flutter by butterfly'
	Didochokinetic rate

Evaluating your assessment with reports from other professionals

The assessment procedures you undertake will provide detailed information on the child's language and will help to isolate the specific areas of deficit for the child concerned. You must, however, evaluate the results of tests performed by other professionals.

The results of *audiological evaluation* are essential to the diagnosis of language deficits in children. The audiologist's report will probably include a description of the assessment procedures that were used for an individual child, the results of the tests and hearing thresholds, if these have been established, and any recommendations that were made. A copy of the audiogram may also be enclosed. It is helpful to know whether the child was able to co-operate with the testing and carry out the test procedures at the level expected for the child's chronological age.

A summary of the procedures most frequently used in routine audiological assessment is given in Table 4.

Table 4 Audiological evaluation: a summary of
recognised procedures

Free field

Test	Age	Method of testing	Information derived
Screening	6–9 months	Sound stimulation of low and high tones within the frequency spectrum. The test stimuli used are 'meaningful' sounds – voice/high-frequency rattle/'S'	Pass–Fail for signals at minimal levels. Hearing levels are not established. Two fails indicate a need for full audiological evaluation

Test	Age	Method of testing	Information derived
Distraction	6–18 months	The child's attention is attracted by one tester in front. When the interest factor is reduced a second tester makes sounds (as above) 3 ft from the child's ear and at an angle of 45° to the child's head	The child has to respond to two low- and two high-frequency 'minimal' signals at each side to pass the tests
Co-operative	18–30 months	As some children of this age inhibit during distraction type tests, the child's growing understanding of language is used. Simple spoken commands are given 3 ft from each ear. High frequencies are tested on 'S' and a high-frequency rattle	In a diagnostic test the level of the signal is raised until the child responds

A careful measure of the levels is made using a sound level indicator |
| *Performance* | 2½–3½ years | The child is conditioned to perform a simple task for 'GO' low-frequency signals and 'S' high-frequency signals. The child must be mature enough to wait, listen and respond | |
| *Pure-tone audiometry* | 3+ years onwards | 1) *Air conduction*: pure tones, particularly within the speech frequency range 250–4000 Hz are tested by the use of an audiometer and headphones | Hearing thresholds are established for each ear giving a measurement of the total hearing system |

Test	Age	Method of testing	Information derived
		2) *Bone conduction*: as above but a vibrator is placed over the mastoid process instead of head-phones 500 Hz/1000 Hz/2000 Hz are the usual frequencies tested	New hearing thresholds are measured and recorded for both ears. Any differences between the air and bone conduction thresholds are a measure of hearing loss attributed to middle-ear problems
		3) *Masking*: When the air conduction thresholds in one ear are better than the other, masking may be necessary. White noise or pure tone is fed into the better ear whilst tests are repeated on the worst ear	The 'true' thresholds for the worst ear are established
Impedance measurement	All ages	The test requires passive co-operation. A probe unit and electra-coustic impedance bridge machine are used	Provides information on middle ear function and is an important measure to establish the presence and nature of a conductive hearing loss
Brain stem and electric response test (BSER)	All ages	This is a measurement of hearing from electrical signals generated by the brain. It provides a measure of the way a subject is responding to sounds and is especially useful for babies and handicapped children who cannot co-operate in conventional tests of	By examining the wave form the tester is able to assess 1) the hearing thresholds for high frequencies generally thought to be about 4000 Hz 2) whether there is any abnormality of the hearing pathway from cochlea to

Speech Discrimination tests

Test	Age	Method of testing and information derived
Kendall Toy Test	2½ years	This test is composed of a selection of toy items – three sets of fifteen toys in each set of which ten items are considered test items and five distractors. The child is required to point to the items named but is not required to speak. The loudness levels of the stimulus words can be monitored on a sound-level indicator.
Word lists	7+ years	These can be either in the free field where the loudness levels of the words spoken can be monitored on a sound-level indicator or by closed circuit (headphones and an adjustable attenuator) using a recorded word list. The listener is asked to repeat what he thinks he hears, even if it is not a recognised word. The word lists are designed to be of equal difficulty – ten words per list. Scoring for each word is out of a maximum of three (one for each syllable). After each list has been completed at a predetermined loudness the percentage of correct utterances is calculated. A curve known as the speech discrimination curve is plotted to show the percentage of syllables scored correctly against loudness. It is usual to plot the speech discrimination curve on the same form as the pure tone audiogram in order to make a simple calculation to determine the degree of correlation between the loss of hearing for pure tones and the loss for speech discrimination.
Manchester Picture Test		This test is used for mentally and linguistically retarded children who cannot undertake the word lists described above. The test is composed of a set of pictures and the child is asked to select a word from a group of items in each picture. No speech is required from the child for this test.

The report from the *psychologist* will usually include information on the tests that were used, together with the information derived from those tests and the recommendations that have been made. The report from the psychologist and/or reports from the *school* will help to identify any additional learning difficulties that may be contributing to the child's language deficit *or* they may confirm that the child's problems are primarily linguistic with normal or above average abilities in other areas of development and learning.

Finally, you should remember that assessment cannot be isolated from remediation. Whilst the major part of your assessment will occur in the initial stages of your contact with the child you will continue to evaluate the child through your treatment programmes.

CHAPTER 4

The developmentally young child: observational assessment procedures

This chapter will consider some of the questions the student should ask when faced with the developmentally immature child or a child where a linguistic framework of description is not appropriate. The aim is to build up a *descriptive profile* of a child's abilities and to estimate the developmental level in areas associated with language acquisition. This form of qualitative assessment does not provide age levels but can be used to describe the problem and form a basis for an intervention programme. The student must know what to look for and how to interpret the observations. An attempt must be made to estimate whether all or some of the child's responses and behaviour can be described as:

approximately age appropriate;

developmentally immature but acceptable in view of an additional handicap, medical history or adverse environmental factors;

atypical and having a detrimental effect on the child's future development or learning.

In order to build up a developmental profile observations must be systematic and based on a sound knowledge of the developmental stages in a given area.

The observational profile in this chapter has been divided into the following sections:

A. Pre-verbal abilities

1.   Socially instigated behaviour
2.   Cognitive and symbolic responses
3.   Attention control
4.   Motor abilities
5.   Elementary comprehension (situational understanding)
6.   Elementary expressive abilities   .

B. Verbal abilities

1.   Verbal comprehension   } emergent language
2.   Verbal expression

The questions and observations are not exhaustive and provide a *guideline* only.

The student is advised to consult recommended textbooks on child development and the checklists summarised in the previous chapter.

After each set of questions and observations in the following profiles, a number of responses are suggested. These are collated into *positive aspects* marked with a plus sign (+) describing behaviour that might be expected as part of normal developmental progress, and *negative aspects*, marked with a minus sign (–) describing behaviour that may indicate abnormal, very delayed or atypical development.

Building up an observational profile

A. Pre-verbal abilities

1. Socially instigated behaviour

Is the child alert and aware of people and objects in his surroundings?

How does the child behave spontaneously?

Does the child initiate and respond to social activities?

Observe

how the child enters the clinic

his willingness to leave his mother and join in activities

his general co-operation with both his mother and the student

obvious signs of affection and response to physical contact

appropriate smiling and laughing

excessive demands for affection or attention

his manner of exploration, degree of curiosity and anticipation

his level of physical activity and ability to ignore distractions

What to do

engage the child in simple activities such as building a tower of bricks, posting objects in a box, an easy form board

---

+ THE CHILD

shows signs of interest and curiosity
explores the room and its contents in a purposeful manner

keeps close to the mother until reassured but then responds to activities initiated by the student *or* co-operates with support from the mother *or* is willing to be enticed into an activity with the student on his own with no separation difficulties

enjoys the attention of a friendly adult, smiles and laughs appropriately, appreciates a humorous situation, shows anticipation when an intriguing event is repeated

shows or offers toys and initiates social responses such as waving goodbye

co-operates willingly, can be controlled by his interest in the activity at least for short periods

– THE CHILD

shows fleeting attention and explores the room in a haphazard manner

is physically very active and restless and/or easily distracted

is aloof, withdrawn and detatched from both his mother and the student

shows *prolonged* reluctance to separate from his mother with signs of distress, marked apprehension, excessive clinging or demands for attention or temper tantrums

rarely looks at mother or student

shows little or fleeting interest in toys

shows little anticipation or curiosity

wanders away from the situation and can only be controlled by physical constraint

may smile or laugh to himself rather than in response to others

may resent physical contact even from a familiar adult but indulge in ritualistic activities such as rocking, spinning or flicking fingers

may show extreme reactions of fear or excitement for no obvious reason

shows apathy and may need an extremely high level of activity on the part of the adult to elicit a response

Remember

that under the age of 2.00 to 2.06 years children are still very dependent on a familiar adult and may resent direct approaches from a stranger. Always be prepared to use the mother to instigate the activities, at least initially in the assessment. Observations on the mother/child interaction can provide very useful data;

that children under 2.00 to 2.06 years have fluctuating attention control and are physically active. Frequent changes of activity are needed and the student should be aware that some of the negative responses may be precipitated through boredom, frustration or fatigue.

2. Cognitive and symbolic responses

What is the level of the child's symbolic understanding?

Does the child demonstrate 'definition by use' of everyday objects?

Does the child demonstrate simple pretend play?

Does the child demonstrate sequenced or imaginative play?

Equipment

Here it is necessary to provide appropriate toys and set up a more structured situation

Everyday objects: cup/spoon/hairbrush/toothbrugh/+ toy telephone/doll/toy car

Large size toys: doll/teddy bear/toy cup and spoon/doll's bed and chair/baby's hairbrush and comb/small toothbrush/doll's dress and shoes/toy telephone

What to do

Provide the child with a selection of everyday objects first and later the large toys

Observe

1) the child's spontaneous response to everyday objects
2) the child's response to the large toys
3) the child's imitation of modelled activities
4) possible improvisation by the child

+THE CHILD

spontaneously demonstrates definition by use by appropriate action, e.g. pretends to drink from the cup/brush his own or his mother's hair/pretends to eat from the spoon imitates definition by use either immediately or later in the session when the activity has been modelled by the mother or student

demonstrates simple pretend play by carrying out appropriate activities on the doll or teddy bear

imitates activities on doll when modelled

demonstrates sequential play by activities such as undressing the doll, putting it to bed then waking it up and feeding it

improvises if appropriate toys are not available, e.g. uses a spatula for a spoon or a comb or toothbrush/makes a cardboard box into a car or bath

pretends actions such as turning on imaginary taps/pouring from an imaginary teapot

imitates imaginary actions and uses them appropriately later in the session

– THE CHILD

shows lack of interest or only fleeting visual inspection of the toys or objects

reacts to the toys in a ritualistic or perseverative manner, e.g. twiddles or spins them or places all toys in a line

shows interest in the toys or objects but at an immature exploratory level, e.g. may mouth, pat, bang or throw but does not use them appropriately

reacts to toys in a destructive manner or becomes involved with one toy only, showing distress if this removed or his 'play' interrupted

cannot be separated from his 'comforter', e.g. blanket, piece of clothing, teddy

imitates *immediately* but does not sustain this or reproduce this at any other time

Remember

During the progression from the exploratory level of play to the representational or pretend level the child may demonstrate a wide variety of actions with the toys. Incidence of appropriate use of objects either by the child himself or with his mother or doll may be fleeting or infrequent and judgements should not be made on one session alone.

In a more formal or structured play session the child may fail to imitate an activity or produce it to order. This does not mean that it is not within his repertoire and he may demonstrate it at a later time or in his own choice of activities.

3. Attention control

What is the child's level of attention control?

(*a*) during his own spontaneous activities?
(*b*) when under adult direction?

What to do

(*a*) allow the child to select a toy or activity of his own choice
(*b*) engage the child in activity preferably one with minimal verbal needs and a high interest or reward value

Equipment

easy construction toys or toys where an activity is involved, e.g. ring stacks/posting boxes/simple form boards

Observe

whether there is fleeting attention and a high level of distraction/ an inability to attend for any length of time even to an activity of the child's own choice

an ability to attend to an activity of his own choice but unable to tolerate interruption without a loss of concentration

an ability to attend to a shared activity but needing considerable control an ability to attend to a shared activity for short periods with minimal adult control

| +THE CHILD |

can occupy himself for short periods and attends to a toy or activity of his own choice to allow for some exploration or action

can *tolerate* a shared activity and when engaged with an adult his attention span can be extended by adult control or intervention

can attend to a shared activity with minimal adult control even if this is for short periods only and frequent changes of activity may be needed

can attend to a task for the reward of completing the task or gaining adult approval

can sustain flexible attention and tolerate interruption

| −THE CHILD |

fails to or rarely occupies himself and his attention is disrupted by his inability to ignore distractions

attends to self-initiated activities but in a ritualistic or obsessional manner and cannot tolerate/accept adult direction

needs physical restraint or very firm adult control before he can attend

is distracted by his own activity and side-tracked by self-induced actions

cannot attend because of anxiety, may be distressed or preoccupied with himself

Remember

There are certain developmental stages in attention control and an observed behaviour may be indicative of an immature level of attention control rather than an abnormal state.

Tasks or activities at an inappropriate developmental level may also lead to disruption of attention control, and the student must be prepared to try a variety of activities with the child in order to establish the child's basic attentional level.

4. Motor abilities

1. *General motor skills*
2. *Specific oral motor skills*

   Although general motor skills are not necessarily directly related to language acquisition, assessment often provides an indication of the overall developmental level of the child

   What level of competence, control and co-ordination has the child achieved in motor skills?

   How does the speech musculature function?

Observe

   (*a*) general posture and mobility/range and co-ordination of motor skills

   watch the child walking/getting on and off a chair/running/going up and down stairs/kicking and catching a ball

   (*b*) manual dexterity/type of grasp/use of both hands/ability to perform an intended movement

   watch the child when he is engaged in simple motoric activities such as brick play/ring stacks/form boards

   (*c*) the general posture of the oro-facial structures at rest and the movements during drinking/eating and spontaneous or elicited attempts to make sounds

   Check with the mother on the general feeding competence. If appropriate watch the child eating a biscuit and drinking .

General motor skills and manual dexterity

+ THE CHILD

is independently mobile and walks with one foot in front of the other/can stop and start safely

can climb on to and get off a chair without aid

can manage stairs independently even though two feet may still be placed on each tread

can run and jump up and down

attempts to kick/throw and catch a ball although the aim may be inaccurate and the end result not achieved

reaches out for objects and toys/uses a prehensile grasp/uses free hand to steady and support when attempting a construction task/ can pick up and release small objects/turns pages of book accurately

can carry out selected movements without excessive overflow

can inhibit associated movements

– THE CHILD

is not independently mobile

is mobile but walks with a wide immature gait/is unsteady/moves in a jerky manner/cannot stop and start at will/appears clumsy/ falls frequently/bumps into furniture/walks on tiptoe most of the time

has difficulty with co-ordinated sequenced movements/cannot manage stairs without adult aid/cannot climb on and off furniture/cannot balance and aim to kick a ball

uses immature palmar grasp/uses only one hand and fails to steady or support objects in a manual activity/cannot pick up or release small objects cannot inhibit associated movements/shows signs of tremor, stiffness, hypotonicity

N.B.
When confronted with a cerebral-palsied child or a child with a marked neuromotor disorder the assessment of posture and motor ability will need to be considerably more detailed and thorough.

Specific oral motor skills

+ THE CHILD
---

can maintain lip closure and control saliva and achieve a build-up of oral air pressure

can chew, bite and swallow without food or fluid escaping from the mouth and without frequent choking

shows symmetry on reflex movements such as smiling

shows no marked postural abnormalities of the tongue and lips and demonstrates a range and variety of movements/may be willing to imitate movements and sounds

---
− THE CHILD
---

shows asymmetry of the facial structure both at rest and during reflex movement

shows abnormal posture of the speech organs and a reduction in the variety, range and co-ordination of the movements of the tongue/lips/soft palate

has problems with the vegetative functions of biting, chewing and swallowing

has problems with the saliva control/has problems initiating and imitating movements

N.B.
Examination of oro-facial structure and assessment of the movements of the speech organs is an essential part of any speech therapy evaluation. The student is referred to Chapter 3 for a detailed assessment procedure and also to Warner, J. (1981).

5. Elementary understanding (responding to speech + additional situational cues or non-verbal cues such as gesture and expression)

Does the child respond to phrases spoken by a well-known adult as part of a familiar routine?

At this level the child is responding to a recognised tonal and rhythm pattern rather than word meaning

Information is obtained from the mother's reporting and by observations of the child's response to the mother's utterance of a much repeated phrase
'Kiss Mummy'
'Clap hands'

Does the child demonstrate situational understanding by recognising words or phrases in a familiar context?

Try to obtain information on the child understanding and obeying simple instructions spoken in context either by the mother or the student
'Put your coat on now'
'Sit down'
'Give . . . . to Mummy'
'Wave bye bye now we're going'

+THE CHILD

attends to the voice and may turn to the speaker, ceasing his own activity turns to his own name or reacts to words such as *'No'* or *'Don't touch'*

carries out the instruction in part or in whole

$\boxed{-\text{THE CHILD}}$

ignores the voice or only responds when a gesture or prompt is used

shows no understanding of familiar, much repeated phrases in a well-established routine

N.B.
Before any estimates of this level of understanding or higher levels of verbal comprehension are made *audiological evaluation is essential*. Whenever possible a hearing test should be carried out before a speech and language assessment is attempted.

6. Elementary expressive abilities
Does the child vocalise to himself and indulge in sound play?

Does the child respond to adult vocalisations and speech by increasing his own vocal and sound play?

Does the child use tuneful vocalisations with stress and cadence patterns to gain attention and 'communicate'?

Observe
the child when he is engaged in his own spontaneous activity or interacting with his mother

Note
the quality and quantity of his vocalisations, particularly the cadences and any consonant/vowel combination

Engage
the child in a simple activity which can be accompanied by short, repetitive phrases which can be said by the adult with slightly exaggerated intonation

e.g. *'in there'* = falling inflection
'another one' = fall/rise inflection
'all gone' = fall/rise inflection

Note

if the child picks up and tries to copy the intonational glides in his vocalisations

Engage

the child in a simple activity and observe whether he vocalises to gain attention or maintain adult interaction in the game

+ THE CHILD

uses a variety of vowel sounds with cadence or consonant/vowel sequences to 'communicate'. These may be accompanied by gesture

increases vocalisations when excited or wanting to gain attention or desired object

uses vowels or simple consonant/vowel sequences imitating the adult intonation glides and stress

– THE CHILD

rarely vocalises except for distress signals

vocalises on vowel sounds but without cadence changes

grunts, pants or makes sounds only by chance such as lip-smacking noises when feeding

makes no direct attempt to vocalise to gain attention

rarely imitates adult model or increases his output in response to adult vocalisation or speech

B. Verbal abilities

1. Verbal comprehension
2. Verbal expression

Once the child can select a particular object in response to an adult request to *find/show me/give me* and is attempting to name, more objective measures of attainment can be introduced and standardised testing may be attempted. The Reynell Developmental Language Scales (1977), revised edition, would be the most suitable test for this stage in development.

However, test scores should be supplemented by additional data obtained from situations where the constraints on the child and student are less rigorous. Here the student can also evaluate the degree of structure and intervention needed in order to plan and carry out successful treatment at this level.

Although it is possible to achieve information on both comprehension and expression with the following suggestions, the student should not *demand* both activites from the child at the same time unless there is clear evidence from spontaneous behaviour that he is ready to follow instructions and talk himself.

Equipment

A box of attractive, fairly large toys containing objects found in early vocabulary of young children
e.g.   car/doll/teddy/cup/shoe/sock/brush/ball/duck/spoon/chair/ clock/dog

What to do

Keep the box on your lap and introduce the toys one at a time. Use facial expressions and phrases such as *'Oh look!'* to maintain attention and anticipation. When three toys are on the table ask the child to *show/find/give me/give Mummy* one of the toys. If necessary help the child with gesture or a physical prompt if he fails. He may need time to learn the task. When one toy has been given replace it with another from the box so that the selection is always one from three.

or

If the child's attention control allows for several toys to be presented at once give him the box and allow him to explore at his leisure. Then ask him to *show/find/give* the toys *or* to help you put them back in the box one at a time when named.

Note

The child's successful selection *and* the errors. Is there confusion of words in a similar semantic category or words that sound alike?

Note

Any spontaneous *naming*: remember that a child may be reluctant to name on demand but is happy to do so in a game situation, particularly if an element of surprise is present, e.g. if the toys are only partly revealed and the child has to 'guess'. This allows for errors to be made without threat as there is no absolute right or wrong answer.

Remember

A child who is reluctant to carry out instructions or has poor motor abilities may 'eye point'. Keep the toys well spread out to allow for this. As this is not a formal test situation requests can be repeated but it is important to note the amount of repetition needed.

Equipment

Make a simple posting box. This is particularly effective if a false bottom can be removed to allow hidden toys to appear or posted toys to reappear.

Collect a selection of smaller toys representing common objects which are suitable for posting.

What to do

Demonstrate the posting activity so that the child understands the game.

Present a few toys at a time and ask the child to post them in the box when named. Remember that a very young child may respond to *'Bye Bye . . . .'* more readily than a longer utterance or instruction. If the child is very eager to post the toys, gently restrain his hands whilst you name the required object.

Note

As above: correct selection of toys and any spontaneous naming.

Remember

Spontaneous naming may occur if the student starts to post a toy but hesitates before dropping the object in the box saying *'Bye Bye'* (pause); Child: *'BALL'*.

or

the child may name more readily when posted objects reappear.

Equipment

Toys which have a simple repetitive activity such as form boards/ring stacks/peg boards/building bricks

What to do

Form boards allow for the selection of objects and for spontaneous or imitated naming.

And note

Toys such as ring stacks and building bricks provide an opportunity to elicit words such as *'more'*, *'all gone'*, *'me'*, *'down'*, *'bang'*. Many children may be more willing to produce these words rather than to name.

Equipment

Toys for doll play, e.g. large-sized bed/chair/cups/brush/spoon.

What to do

Engage the child in doll play and include simple instructions such as *'Make dolly sleep'*, *'Give dolly a drink'*, *'Brush dolly's hair'*.

Note

Successful response to instructions and any spontaneous words especially ones that may not be direct naming of the objects, e.g. *'drink'/juice/milk'* rather than *'cup'*.

Tape recording

Each session should be tape recorded so that all spontaneous speech is available for analysis later. With the child functioning at an immature attention level it is impossible to write and engage and control the child at the same time. The student should note any words used, estimate whether these were spontaneous/imitated or echoed and also note intonation, stress and sound patterns.

Comprehension

| +THE CHILD |

selects named objects in response to the student's/mother's request

indicates an understanding of the word by eye pointing or a hand movement towards the object without fully completing the instruction

responds to the instruction but needs additional information such as *'where's the brush'* = no response, *'you know the one you do your hair with'* = correct response

| −THE CHILD |

demonstrates random selection of objects with no clear evidence that the *word* is understood, may respond some of the time if a gesture is used with the verbal request

selects one object consistently, e.g. car but shows no understanding of other requests for objects.

Expression

+THE CHILD

produces spontaneous consistent attempts at words *'ba'* for *'ball'* *'me'*, *'more'*

or

produces a specific name, e.g. *'Pi'* (Prince) for dog

imitates or attempts to imitate the student or mother/uses words + jargon cadences

─THE CHILD

makes no attempt to name or imitate/remains virtually silent or makes random sounds without cadence or stress

demonstrates echoic imitation of whole utterance or the beginning or end of an utterance

Drawing inferences from observational data

Observational data do not provide exact age levels but do attempt to describe the normal and abnormal behaviours that may be encountered at any age in the more damaged or developmentally immature child. They do not replace differential diagnosis but rather give guidance for the more detailed aspects of treatment.

In children progressing through the normal developmental processes, however slowly, one would expect to find a higher proportion of positive responses and behaviour. Negative responses may still be seen as part of the developmental progress from immaturity towards maturity. They may also be evoked by stress or inappropriate handling. With the more damaged child or the child where development is severely retarded the proportion of negative responses is likely to be significantly greater. Even with these children some positive responses will be observed if a developmental baseline is established through careful and thorough assessment. These positive responses may also be increased with appropriate management.

Following the assessment it is necessary to consider what form of treatment or management would be most appropriate for an individual child. If sufficient evidence has been collected from the assessment to support the hypothesis that the child is passing through the normal developmental stages, but at a slower rate, *direct* intervention may not be required. It may be necessary to provide the parents with an explanation of the problem, to give support and practical guidance in handling the child at a realistic developmental level. Regular reviews and reassessment will be required to monitor progress and intervention may be needed at a later stage if progress is not maintained or additional problems arise.

If one particular aspect of development shows a slower rate of progress than the others, an intervention programme may have to be instigated to encourage and develop that ability and bring it in to line with the overall developmental level.

Where behaviour is markedly abnormal the therapeutic programme may have to focus on a reduction of the atypical responses in order to allow future learning to take place. A specific intervention programme may have to be designed for the child, based initially on behaviour modification techniques. This programme must take into account the needs of the parents or caregivers and be one that can be followed outside the clinical environment.

CHAPTER 5

The developmentally young child: management and treatment

The creative process of therapeutic intervention will be influenced in all aspects by the people involved. The child's individual needs and strategies will dictate the nature and timing of the intervention. The therapist's personality will greatly influence the manner in which all procedures are carried out. The following chapter describes activities which have proved to be helpful in many cases. It will be up to the student to determine which measures will be useful in any one case. She must then find out how to apply them so that they become part of her own therapeutic repertoire.

Successful intervention depends on establishing the degree and nature of control needed by the child in order for him to learn and in creating a variety of appropriate activities to facilitate learning. The student clinician has to learn to alter and adapt her manner and approach to suit the individual child's needs.

The student may be confronted by:

The willing participant:
here the child's attention and co-operation is governed predominantly by the interaction created between the child and the adult. The need for direct discipline is minimal and control is maintained by judicious choice of activities and the reduction of frustration and boredom. The adult's role is one of support and guidance. Considerable flexibility and ingenuity may be needed to maintain the momentum for the child but the adult is free to follow the child's lead and to use the child's own choice of activity.

The disruptive child:
here the child is unable to co-operate easily of his own volition. A high level of adult participation is required and the child needs the adult to control his behaviour for him and direct him in order for learning to take place. The adult is less free to follow the child's lead and may have to *structure* both the environment and the activities.

The reluctant participant:
here the child's level of co-operation is restricted by his level of apprehension. The child may manifest his anxiety by a reluctance to commit himself to any activity. Direct demands for participation should not be made initially. The approach should be supportive and friendly, but not effusive and the attention and interest should be created on the activity rather than the child. Care should be taken to select a task that is well within the child's level of competence so that success is guaranteed when the child is ready to join in.

The manipulative child:
here the child will resort to a variety of behaviours to get his own way and avoid participating. He may demand attention by pretending to cry, sulking, taunting the adult by deliberate 'naughty' behaviour, refusing to co-operate in tasks he has previously enjoyed or clinging to his mother. Experience will help the student recognise this situation and every effort should be made to discover why the child resorts to this form of behaviour. The student should try to avoid direct confrontation with the child and adopt a fairly detached manner. Persuasion and cajoling rarely work and again the interest and attention should be placed on the task not the child.

The apathetic child:
here the child is very passive and shows little interest in his surroundings or in initiating activities. The apathetic child is not difficult to control but demands a high level of adult input

and energy before a response can be obtained. Physical prompts may have to be used initially in order to activate the child. Care should always be taken not to confuse apathy with apprehension as it can be seen that a very different approach is needed in each case.

The student should also remember that physical handicap will place additional constraints on both the child and the adult. Interaction may involve more physical contact and manipulation. Where physical contact is a necessary part of the therapeutic programme the student must handle the child in a confident but gentle manner, never surprise the child by sudden action and always make sure the child is comfortable and in a position which allows maximum co-operation.

Management

Structuring the environment

Whenever possible try to reduce the level of distraction in the room. Put unwanted toys and expensive equipment away and, when you can, lock cupboard doors.

Plan ahead and have the toys and equipment for your session looked out before the child arrives. Keep the materials for the session by your side in a large box or bag so that you can introduce one activity at a time. Clear up each activity before introducing a new one. It is very difficult for a child to attend selectively if the floor or table is covered with toys. Too many toys may also precipitate exploration or inspection rather than play or the desired response to a task.

Decide on your work space. If you choose the floor, make sure the child cannot hurt himself on big furniture. Although small children play naturally on the floor it is sometimes easier to control the situation and focus attention by working at a small table.

With a very active or restless child, position the table and chair in such a way as to minimise the child's escape route. Place the child's chair against the wall and position yourself on one side and the mother on the other. Remember that it may be very difficult to get a child to return to the work space once he has left and it is easier to keep control if the child's space is restricted for some of the time.

If the child tends to use his mother as a refuge or turns to her constantly for assistance when it is not really needed, seat her close to the child at first, until he is used to you and the room and then gradually move her chair further away. Remember that an anxious mother may interrupt the interaction between you and the child, either by physical means or by a flow of verbal instructions. If this happens reassure the mother, explain what you are trying to achieve and gently tell her to let you find out how the child responds to you on his own.

Some very young children work better when sitting on their mother's knee or standing close to her. If this does not interfere with the child's co-operation, allow it to happen. The child will usually separate and sit down without a fuss once he is confident or intrigued.

Controlling the situation

Try to establish a pattern for the onset of each session. A child responds to a familiar routine. Teach him your 'rules' — *'when we play with the toys we sit at the table'/'before we get another toy this one must go back in the box'*.

If the more difficult child has an activity he enjoys, try introducing this as a 'reward' when he has completed an activity of your choice. Help him understand *'That was very good. Now we can play with the football/toy telephone'. 'We've had my game/ toy now you can choose the game/toy'*. Try to avoid introducing the toy too early in the session as it may then be difficult to wean the child from the toy or attract his attention with other materials.

If a child is obsessed with one particular toy you may either have to keep it out of sight or, if the child refuses to settle without it, produce it to avoid precipitating a distress response. Part of your future therapy will be to introduce an activity for the child to complete before he has the desired toy. This may have to be a very simple task at first and one that only takes a short time, e.g. putting a mannikin in a boat/ a ring on a stack/a peg in a board. The aim is then to increase the length and complexity of the task, gradually, before producing the toy.

When planning therapy to increase attention or co-operation, remember that the *task* is not the important thing. It is the child's response and reaction that should be the focus as you are not trying to teach a manipulative skill. Choose a simple activity that is well within the child's level of competence and one that has a quick reward. Give the child clear directions, either by verbal means if he understands or by demonstration. Reinforce a desired response immediately so that the child knows that he has done well or what was expected of him. Try, whenever possible, to use social or verbal reinforcement. Remember to increase the demands on the child gradually. Once he has gained a short-term goal lengthen the space between your reinforcements.

Example

The child is required to put the mannikins back in a wooden boat, one after the other without intervening activity or distraction.

Step 1

Give the child *one* mannikin, help him with a physical prompt if necessary, to put the mannikin in the boat. When he has done this smile/clap your hands/say *'Good'*. Repeat if necessary.

Step 2

Give the child *one* mannikin to put back on his own without help. When he has done this reward him as above. Repeat if necessary.

Step 3

Give the child one mannikin, when this has been put in the boat, hand him another — say *'and another one'*; delay the praise until there are two mannikins in the boat. Repeat with another *two* mannikins.

Step 4

Repeat as for step 3 but do not praise until the child has put *three* mannikins back, then *four*.

Step 5

Expect *all* the mannikins to be put in the boat before you praise or reward.

Remember

that if you introduce a new activity such as rings on a stack, you may have to praise or reward for each ring at first.

Controlling and helping the child

If the child is unable or reluctant to join in there are a number of strategies that can be tried.

Become *involved* in the activity or play yourself, look as though it is fun and interesting. Do not make direct demands on the child and do not pivot your attention on him when he joins in. Make sure the toys are within his reach and include him in a relaxed and easy way.

Remember a child will often do something through a third person such as a teddy bear or doll. *'Let's make teddy put the car in the box'* may work better than direct demands for the child's co-operation.

Use the mother or sibling to demonstrate. Say *'Mummy try. Put the little man in the boat. That's good'*. The child will then often join in of his own volition. Again do not focus your attention on him directly at first.

A challenge sometimes works well, say *'I bet you don't know where the cup is'*.

Modelling is also important for the child. Demonstrate the activity first for the child and then take turns. For example, when using an object form board say *'I'm taking out the ball'* (pretend to search for and find the correct piece). Then invite the child to have a turn. Let him choose his own object to remove at first and then gradually ask him to find ones named by you.

Always remember to *show* a child what is required of him. Do not rely on verbal understanding until you have good evidence a child can follow instructions.

Follow the child's lead. Children under the age of 2–2½ years tend to be naturally self-willed. It may be more successful to intervene in the child's own activity rather than try to superimpose one against the child's inclination. With ingenuity most activities can be turned into a language-learning game. Remember, however, that at some stage you will have to direct the child towards your choice of activity in order to help him acquire skills he may not have. Demonstration and involving yourself in the activity may be the best form of enticement.

Do not be afraid to be firm and to use gentle physical restraint when needed. For example placing your hands over the child's to reduce fiddling whilst you give an instruction *or* putting an arm on the child's chair to stop him pushing it back or rocking it. Avoid direct physical confrontation and a 'tussle', but remember that you may have to collect the child from the other side of the room and return him firmly to the task. Use a 'no nonsense' approach by remaining involved but a little detached. Physical prompts can be used in order to keep a child's attention and involvement.

If the child suddenly becomes unco-operative or fretful try a change of activity as a distraction technique.

If the child is unco-operative and deliberately trying to disrupt the situation, try ignoring him and *either* put all the toys away in an unemotional manner and wait quietly until he returns or is willing to join in *or* concentrate on the activity or play rather than the child. This routine is only effective in a room where there are few additional attractions for the child.

Ride out temper tantrums by being calm and slightly detached. Once the tantrum is over return to the game/toy/activity in a quiet and welcoming way. Remember that a child needs time to recover from an outburst and will need your reassurance and support when it is all over.

Remember too that the mother may feel very anxious, distressed or embarrassed by her child's behaviour. Tell her what your policy is: *'Let's leave him alone for a moment. He can't cope with pressure for a while'* . . . *'Don't worry, let him get over it and I'll try again'.* Your uncritical and calm attitude will help to reassure the mother and prevent a worsening situation.

Sometimes temper tantrums/rage/sudden refusals can be a good sign especially in a child who is usually apathetic or detached. It is important to let the mother know that her child's apparent immature behaviour may be the first sign of real awareness or contact.

If all else fails the child can be removed from the situation by taking him from the room. This must be done in an impersonal and unemotional manner and the child should not be returned to the room until he has calmed down. Do not use this technique if the child is trying to manipulate his own escape.

Remember that certain behaviours may be developmentally appropriate for an individual child and he may react to toys at that level. For example, the child may still be at the 'throwing' stage with toys. If you do not obtain evidence of more advanced levels of play, either spontaneously or in imitation, it is inappropriate to demand a higher level of interaction. It is important to work at the child's level and to find ways of extending his responses. (See following section on treatment methods.)

Some children do not like direct physical contact and retreat or show distress when touched. This response is usually more marked for light casual touch and the child may react favourably to 'rough' play, such as tickling, bouncing or being jumped up and down. Care should be taken to establish whether physical contact is acceptable and if so what form the child will tolerate. With the child who reacts adversely to casual touch this should be avoided in the early stages of treatment and introduced gradually in appropriate situations such as washing hands.

Where physical contact is an essential part of treatment, the child must be handled with confidence. Physically handicapped children may protest and cry but the student should not be perturbed by the child's response and continue working in a firm but humorous manner.

The extremely shy or apprehensive child may be easily threatened by too much enthusiasm and a high level of adult participation. The more extroverted student may have to curb an outgoing manner until the child can tolerate a lively approach to therapy.

The apathetic or passive child conversely requires a high energy output on the part of the adult and may need a more forceful and directive manner before a response can be obtained. A positive and dynamic approach must be taken.

Treatment

The following treatment suggestions are directed towards the child needing help at a pre-verbal level or the child needing help with early, emergent language.

Intervention may need either to consolidate emerging skills and help the child become proficient at his own level, or to act as a directive to advance the child's own abilities in any given area.

Treatment may be concerned with one or more of the following:

1. Early social development and basic interaction

2. Attention control to enable the child to benefit from environmental stimulation and experience and to acquire some degree of self-direction

3. Concept formation and symbolic understanding to expand the child's knowledge of his world

4. Situational and contextual understanding to facilitate verbal comprehension

5. Imitation of action and sounds to form the foundation for verbal expressive abilities

Points to note

Toys and games are chosen as a vehicle of learning and one toy or game may be used in a variety of ways to teach differing skills. It is important to establish that the child knows the 'rules of the game', however simple, before any additional demands are made. A child can only learn one new thing at a time. Before introducing your ideas or objectives, allow the child to have time to explore a toy. This will also give you time to see what the child does on his own and to decide whether you can use this to achieve your treatment aim.

The structure and objective for each activity must be clear in your own mind but it is important to remember that the way a child reaches an objective will vary with the individual child's responses and abilities. This demands both careful planning and a high degree of flexibility.

Therapy will only be successful if it is absorbed into the overall management of the child. Parent or caregiver participation is essential and a student may be asked by the clinician in charge to assume the role of parent adviser as part of the intervention programme. Although this may seem a little daunting at first, it is important to remember that parents learn more from observing the clinical session than from long explanations. The student may have to prepare a written programme for the parents to take home and must be ready to answer questions but should always consult the therapist if the parents seek advice on matters other than the programme.

The suggestions in the following section are meant as a guide only. The student is advised to get additional ideas from the many books available on toys and play. Experience of working with developmentally immature children will help you build up your own ideas and develop your own style and approach.

Treatment suggestions

Social games

EQUIPMENT
You and the child
or
You and the child + simple 'toys' such as building bricks/cotton reels/cardboard boxes/cotton-wool/kitchen foil/soft ball/rattle/a string of wooden beads/Kelly doll.

OBJECTIVES
Eliciting early social responses and establishing a 'dialogue' between you and the child.

Establishing a shared frame of reference.

Attracting and holding attention for a short moment.

Mediating between the child and an object/toy.

Stimulating: watching/curiosity/anticipation.

Encouraging vocal conversations.

Responding to activity initiated by the child and influencing the timing and content of what the child is doing.

WHAT TO DO

Keep the child so that face-to-face contact or play is possible.

React in varying ways such as smiling/showing surprise or delight to any gesture or overture from the child. Alter your timing by delaying the response, encourage repetition by turning your face away and peeping round suddenly.

Encourage the child to receive and proffer toys in simple 'giving and taking' games.

Make a game out of any spontaneous action by the child such as throwing or dropping toys. Again alter your timing and response/ show anticipation. Try to get the child to throw the object towards you and then make a game of pushing or rolling it back.

Build towers of bricks and either encourage the child to knock the tower down or do this yourself, altering your timing and response.

Play 'peek-a-boo' games with your own face or gently hiding the child's face.

Make toys or objects appear suddenly from unexpected places such as your pocket/under a box. Pretend to hide a toy in one place and make it reappear from somewhere else.

Engage the child's visual attention with mobile or mechanical toys.

Engage the child's auditory attention with sound-making toys.

Imitate the child's activity or sounds — make this into a 'your turn—my turn' game or a conversation.

Introduce a variety of materials such as kitchen foil/tissue paper/ string of wooden beads/rattle/Kelly doll, and encourage the child to explore them. See if you can get the child to change his actions according to the material, for example crumple the foil/tear the tissue paper/rock the Kelly doll/shake the rattle.

Encourage simple gestures such as waving bye bye/blowing a kiss.

Action games

EQUIPMENT
You + child and things to climb on, hide behind, open or shut
or
You + child and simple action toys such as large, soft ball/ wooden or plastic car which runs easily/pop-up cone tree.

OBJECTIVES
Sharing physical activity.

Increasing the space between you and the child to allow for less direct control and contact.

Introducing an element of delay before certain actions occur to lengthen attention span.

Encouraging interactive imitation.

Linking action and words to clarify comprehension.

Requesting vocalization or a word before an action or event occurs.

WHAT TO DO
Join in the child's spontaneous physical actions — help him to climb on a low chair, hold your hands and jump off/hide behind the desk for you to find/hold your hand and run to the table — to the door.

As you join in, provide a simple commentary on what is happening to link actions and words — *'up on the chair — hold my hands — now jump down'* (this technique is particularly effective with the very active child who finds it difficult to sit still *or* the passive child who needs rousing and stimulating).

Later

Introduce a pause before an action or event and request a vocalisation or a word before the event occurs

Play kicking/throwing/rolling games with the ball. This is good for attention direction − use simple instructions: *'Look here's the ball'. Later* use this situation to elicit words − *'Who wants the ball?'* ... *'ME'/'What shall I do?'* ... *'KICK'*. Show a car and a ball and ask *'Which one?'* ... *'BALL'*.

Play pushing games with a car, then give a choice from a car or lorry. Repeat the simple questions as above.

Encourage the child to imitate your actions.

Use the pop-up cone tree − help the child at first to stack the cones and set the spring − show him how to make the cones pop up − say *'Look ... Pop'. Later* delay the release of spring until the child says *'POP'*.

Paste pictures on large cardboard cubes − encourage the child to toss these or turn them round on a rod. Name the picture and later take turns and encourage the child to imitate you naming.

Hiding games

EQUIPMENT
Cardboard boxes/cartons/empty yoghurt-pots/cardboard or plastic tube/posting box.

An assortment of correctly sized toys and common objects such as toy brush/cup/spoon/shoe/small bear or doll/horse/car.

Cloth bag with a draw string and a hole large enough to invite the child's hand.

Marble run or toy with several exits.

OBJECTIVES
Enticing the child to explore.

Encouraging the concept of object permanence.

Lengthening attention span by demanding searching and waiting techniques.

Introducing one object at a time with an element of surprise to facilitate early comprehension and naming.

Matching objects to pictures.

WHAT TO DO
Let the child see you hiding the toy or object under one of two boxes or cartons. Encourage him to find it — show surprise — name the toy as it is found.

As above but do not let the child see which box/carton you choose. Ask *'Where's the toy?'* Help the child search by pretending yourself. Name the toy when it is found.

Introduce three or four boxes and hide only one object at first, help the child search and again name. *Later* hide two different objects and ask the child to find one.

Let the child feel for toys in a cloth bag. At first have a variety of the same toys in the bag. This is good for providing repetition for comprehension or naming. When appropriate this game can be used to elicit two-word utterances: *'What have you found?'* ... *'Another car'*. Introduce a variety of objects in the bag and encourage spontaneous or imitated naming as the child produces each object. Put your hand in the bag, ask *'What have I found?'* See if the child can guess. Sometimes make deliberate mistakes and misname; this may encourage simple negative statements from the child.

Use a post box to encourage comprehension. At first place one object in front of the child for him to post when named. Use a physical prompt if necessary. *Later* introduce a choice of one from two then one from three. Make sure the child has one familiar object when introducing a new one, for example, cup (known): add shoe/cup and shoe (known): add car.

Post toys down a cardboard tube and name them as they fall out. Encourage the child to post and later to name for himself.

Remember that both post boxes and post tubes are good for encouraging two-word phrases later, for example: *'bye bye car'/ 'car gone'/'in there'/'here 'tis'*.

Use a marble run or a toy where objects can appear from differing exits. These games are good for encouraging looking and increasing attention. *Later* they can be used to encourage vocalisation, imitation, and elicit phrases such as *'here it is'/'that's a car'*.

Paste pictures on boxes and hide a similar toy under or in the box. Encourage the child to look for the object. When he has found it point to the picture and say *'Here's a car'*, then point to his toy and say *'like your car'*.
Later ask the child to put the object you name in a box with a similar picture.

Action—word games

EQUIPMENT
Inset form boards.

Wooden boat with mannikins.

Ring stacks.

Nesting cups.

Simple constructional toys such as peg boards/locking bricks/ Leggo.

Tupperware alphabet bricks.

OBJECTIVES
Increasing attention control for part of the task leading to the child eventually completing the task for its own sake.

Encouraging comprehension of names and later contextual phrases such as *'give me'/'in there'/'on top'/'push it in'*.

Eliciting imitation of vocalisations with cadence if words are not possible.

Creating a situation which encourages spontaneous speech from the child.

WHAT TO DO
All these games are good for increasing attention span and co-operation. Use the procedure described in *Controlling the situation*.

Object form boards can be used for early comprehension by playing *'find the cat/ball/shoe'*. Setting the insets back helps the understanding of simple contextual phrases such as *'turn it round'/'try another place'*. Use gesture at first if needed.
Put the insets out on the table where the child can see them but not reach them. This encourages imitation or naming as the child has to ask for the one he wants.
Later the form board can be used to elicit phrases such as *'in there'/'cat there'/'cat in'/'fits now'/'no fit'*.

Peg boards/ring stacks/building bricks/simple construction toys can all be used to facilitate the understanding of simple phrases and elicit imitation of sounds, words or phrases, for example *'(it) goes there'/'another one now'/'more bricks'*.
Later these activities can be used to encourage spontaneous speech by delaying the response until the child has asked for a part or told you what to do.

Tupperware alphabet bricks are good for attracting attention. These cubes are designed to open and shut, are brightly coloured and the hidden objects inside rattle. Use them for imitation games and later to elicit appropriate phrases or words *'Which colour do you want, a red brick or a blue brick?' 'RED BRICK'. 'What shall I do now?' 'OPEN THAT ONE'*.

Symbolic understanding and pretend play

EQUIPMENT

Collect a set of life-size or large-toy-size everyday objects. Have two of each object, one for you to model with, one for the child. Choose action toys such as hairbrushes/toothbrushes/cups/spoons/toy telephone/toy iron.

Rag dolls and teddy bears.

Doll's bed/chair/table/bath/cups/spoons/plates.

OBJECTIVES

Facilitating object recognition and symbolic understanding.

Developing a give-and-take routine and imitative interaction.

Providing a situational framework for verbal understanding.

Creating activities that encourage both the naming of objects and actions.

WHAT TO DO

Provide the child with the large objects and model appropriate actions, for example, pretend to drink/eat/brush your hair. Concentrate on the play and actions not the child. Make the play slightly exaggerated by smacking your lips/sipping loudly. Do not force the child to copy – imitation takes time. If the child does not attempt to imitate your actions use physical prompts from time to time *or* carry out the actions on the child.

Respond appropriately if the child carries out the actions on you.

Model actions on a doll or teddy bear. Tell the child: *'Look Dolly's sleeping/eating'*. Invite the child to do the same, *'Make your dolly sleep'*.

Introduce new toys (teddy bear/rabbit/monkey). Through play and modelling show the child that actions can be carried out by different toys, for example, Teddy sleeps/Dolly sleeps/Bunny sleeps. This provides a natural setting for language work on subject change and verb change. *Later* sentence object change can be shown by creating situations where the dolly eats a biscuit/banana/sweet.

Make the play lively and dramatic. Introduce the ridiculous or unexpected sometimes to attract attention.

Later model sequenced play by creating situations where the dolly undresses — washes her face — cleans her teeth and goes to bed.

Make a picture book containing single-page pictures of the objects used in the doll play and the actions. Show the book to the child and say, *'Look here's a cup'*. Help the child turn the pages and find the correct pictures. Delay your own naming of the pictures and see if the child tries to name spontaneously.

Later introduce less realistic materials for imaginative play.

Making and drawing
EQUIPMENT
Collect a 'making box' with paper/glue/sellotape/squares of coloured sticky paper/cotton reels/match boxes/scraps of material and wool/plasticine.

WHAT TO DO
Use your imagination and make a simple toy for the child. Tell him what you are doing. Do not demand co-operation from the child, let him watch and join in if he wishes.

This technique is very good with the apprehensive or reluctant child as it takes the focus from the child and makes you the active partner. It is also excellent later as a framework for language learning.
For example:
comprehension of *actions*: cutting/squeezing/sticking;
illustrating *adjectives*: big/red/round/long/fat;
introducing *nouns*: wheels/door/driver.

Making something for the child is also good at the stage of forced alternatives by introducing choice: *'Shall I give this man blue trousers or red trousers?'*

Draw pictures on the spot for the child even if your drawing is poor. This is often more successful than providing ready-made pictures as it allows the child to see details as they happen. Describe what you are drawing. *'Here's the face – now I'm going to draw the hair – look it's very long – now I'm going to draw the eyes – look my man has blue eyes and a big nose and a mouth and lots of teeth'*.

Make push-pull pictures for the child or tactile pictures by using material/cotton-wool. These pictures are good for later comprehension work and can be taken home by the child to give him something to talk about.

CHAPTER 6

Early speech development: assessment and intervention

Once again the student is reminded that the following procedures have been evolved from the clinical experience of other people. You must therefore guard against following them too slavishly since this could impede the development of your own clinical style. You must also seek to associate them with your overall treatment rationale so that they become integrated into a therapeutic programme.

In this chapter we will consider the child whose language is delayed beyond normal limits but who is able to offer enough speech for an analysis of linguistic features to be carried out. This child will be using this speech as his primary means of communication. Thus the student has material to work on rather than having to stimulate every aspect of language function. The purpose of the analysis has already been indicated and we are here concerned with the practicalities.

The student must conduct her session so as to stimulate and encourage the child to produce his best effort. If this is achieved there will be a speech sample yielded which will indicate the child's present linguistic position and the immediate therapeutic goals. Equally important is the encouragement that the child and his mother may receive from hearing his speech. This may lead to increased attention in the home to speech attempts and the behaviour and conditions that bring them forth.

The following notes are set out to show how sample utterances may be facilitated. It is not possible to establish the meaning underlying the structure. For full appreciation of the meaning which engenders linguistic attempt and is conveyed by its structure, the student must refer to her language texts. For the correct inference to be drawn in any one case she must study not only the literature but the child. These notes are offered to guide the student in conveying to the child the idea that speech influences people and events. As he absorbs and acts upon this premise he will produce his own utterances. While he is making the connection the student may have to offer him several linguistic forms through which he can convey his ideas.

The notes also suggest how the student can build on what the child is offering. Assessment will show her whether intervention is necessary. But in the early stages assessment and treatment must proceed at the same time. The speech or behaviour must be facilitated if the assessment is to be made. Any remedial activity which ensues will only be appropriate if it is carried out with a clearly defined purpose and supported by study of the background literature.

In helping a child to grasp the nature of language it is sometimes necessary to use forms which are not part of the adult language system. A very reduced utterance can help a child with limited memory to hold on to the essential features. Where such structures are suggested they are intended to be used judiciously and never to be the target of rigorous behaviour-modification approaches. Artificial linguistic constructions can have a part to play in the overall clinical theme, which *is always to support and never to extinguish a young child's tentative attempts at spoken language*.

Combining assessment and treatment

When the child offers tentative or infantile utterances in the form of:

> single words,
> two-word combinations,
> words combined with jargon,

first assessment should reveal whether there is a language delay either simple or severe, or whether the limited utterance indicates a major problem in learning the spoken word *or* in learning any symbolic system.

Simple delays should respond to *Language stimulation.*

Severe delays may respond to *Language stimulation* or may require *Language teaching.*

Major learning problems are likely to require *Language teaching* in an environment specially adapted or structured for the purpose.

Simple and severe delays

In cases of simple or severe delay the underlying supposition is that the child has the ability to extract the content and the form of language from his environment. The student should, therefore, highlight features of normal speech to interest and encourage him but should not alter the way in which she uses speech except to:

Reduce length of her utterance to promote listening and imitation.

Reduct rate of her utterance to allow for comprehension and interjection.

Use repetition to increase the clarity of the verbal impression and to assist retention.

If the child is delayed in comprehension the student should give plenty of opportunity for listening to clear and vivid speech.

If the child is delayed in comprehension but maintains the expected comprehension to expression ratio the student should conduct the session so that both speakers have equal opportunity.

If the child is very much delayed in output in relation to comprehension the student should keep her own speech to a minimum and increase the child's opportunities for utterance.

When stimulating speech it is rarely wise to aim for length and clarity at the same time. Techniques to improve clarity may be incorporated into every session but should not be used when the child is trying to increase the amount of speech he uses because of memory strain and conflict.

Procedure
Choose simple toys which do not take time to assemble as the emphasis should be on speech and language work.

Elaborate mechanical toys should be avoided as the child will concentrate on the activity and speech yield may be nil.

Complicated games should be avoided as they take too much time to set up so speech yield may be very low.

Pictures may not be helpful except to increase speed of labelling; however, they are very useful for comprehension development.

Family photographs are particularly valuable for this purpose.

Ideal toys are those which are simple in construction and have several purposes, for example, a wooden boat with mannikins — which may yield such utterances as:

in boat; man in;
more men; red man;
my turn;
man in boat;
more red men;
boat on water.

Adult speech input
This may have two aims but should not attack both at one time.

(a) to increase understanding:
Where's the man?   I'm going to put the little
                                    green man in my boat

Where's the little man?	The little red man is waiting for his turn
Where's the little green man?	Shall we let the green man stay in too? No, the green man's getting out – he's finished his turn.

(b) to encourage modelling and imitation:

Where's man	in boat
Here's man	man in
Here's boat	more in
	push boat
	jump out

Child's output

This may be achieved in the form of responses to (*a*) or in imitation of (*b*). It may also be specifically induced by activities designed to elicit pivot/open class constructions.

Give the child a series of objects so that he can say:

Man in boat	Or	*Man go in*	Or	*My man*
Boy in boat		*Boy go in*		*My boy*
Pussy in boat		*Pussy go in*		*My pussy*

Or	*Man jump*	Or	*Man in there*
	Boy jump		*Boy in there*
	Pussy jump		*Pussy in there*

Try to avoid staying for too long with one construction so as not to induce stereotyped utterances. Once the words are being used move on to other constructions.

Modelling and expansion

These types of responses show children moving at a different rate. The student must alter the amount of information she gives the child according to the level of his response.

STUDENT: 'I'm putting the ball back'

CHILD: *'Me ball'* or *'ball back'*

'You're putting your ball back'

'I'm putting the car back'

   'Car back'

'I'm putting the brick back'

   'Brick back'

   'Allgone'

'Bricks have all gone'

   'Allgone brick'

'Cars have all gone'

   'Allgone car'

   'Me ball back'

'You're putting your ball back in the box'

'I'm putting the car back in the box'

   'Me car back' or *'Me car back no'*

'You're not going to put your car back'

   'Car box no'

'You don't want to put your car in box?'

   'Me table'

'You're leaving your car on the table'

Questioning and Expansion

STUDENT: 'Where's the dog?'

CHILD: *'There'*

'There it is'

'Where's the cat?'

   'There'

'There it is'

'Where's the pig?'

   'There'

'There it is'

'Where's the chicken?'

   'There 'tis'

'There it is. There's the chicken'

   'Floor'

'The dog's on the floor'

'Where's the cat?'

   'On floor'

'The cat's on the floor too. Where's the pig?'

   'Pig on floor'

'The dog and the cat and the pig are all on the floor'

'Where's the chicken?'

   'Box'

'The chicken's in the box, he's not on the floor'

The question demands a little more from the child than does modelling. The student must be highly sensitive to any change which indicates that the child is ready to move on.

The decision as to which technique to use is not determined by the linguistic level but by the character and disposition of the child. Modelling works better with the compliant. With the more individualistic other approaches may be more productive.

Forced alternatives

STUDENT: 'Do you want the little dog or the big dog?'

CHILD: *'Dog'*

'Do you want the pig or the cat?'

   'Cat'

'Do you want the chicken or the cow?'

   'Cow'

'Do you want the big cow or the little cow?'

   'Big'

'Here's the big cow. Now do you want the big horse or the little horse?'

   'Big horse'

   'Big dog'

'Do you want the big black dog or the big brown dog?'

   'Black dog'

'Do you want the dog that's running or the one that's sitting down?'

   'Dog running'

'Here's the big black dog running. Is he running after the sheep or the cat?'

'Sheep'

'And what are the sheep doing? running away or are they fighting?'

'Sheep run away'

The purpose of the forced alternative is to show that a selected speech response is required. It should, therefore, only be employed when the student has evidence that the child has more than one response available to him.

The speed with which the child responds to a lead and moves on will show how accessible words are to him. A swift and regular response by single words suggests that the child is ready for a higher level of performance. So the student should move ahead to demand two words. If he has difficulty in moving from one to two words give him plenty of practice in saying his single words at speed.

Activities

Play 'echo'   Use a puppet or doll and let him say the word first for the child to repeat. Then let the child say the word. Point to the object that the child is to say.

Take objects out of a box while the child names them.

Let the child guess what is in the box.

Deal out picture cards while child names them.

Let him deal while you name. Then he must ask for them.

With both these activities you can keep trying to model two word combinations in case the child is ready to pick them up.

Accompany all such activities with plenty of memory training.

STUDENT: 'The puppet wants you to pick him up and put him down next to Teddy as soon as he waves his hand.
The puppet wants you to find his red coat with the buttons'

(using picture cards)

'Puppet wants car and dog'
'Puppet wants pig and cow'

If the child enjoys the last activity try getting him to ask for two pictures using 'and' to link them.

If the child is able to make use of 'and', consolidate it by showing pictures of 'Mummy and Daddy' or the child and his brother. If no photographs can be found make quick pin-men drawings.

If the child is moving slowly take time to consolidate the two-word utterances.

STUDENT: 'Is that your Mummy or my Mummy?'
CHILD: *'My Mummy'*
'Is she with your Daddy or my Daddy?'
CHILD: *'My Daddy'*

Make pin-men drawings to show Mummy walking and Daddy sitting and Mummy pushing the pram and Daddy carrying the baby etc. Use appropriate stress and intonation with all utterances to assist the child's memory. If he cannot name the whole activity let him supply one or two of the words.

If the child moves swiftly into using two- or three-word utterances, increase the amount and kind of material to stimulate use of adverbs, adjectives, verbs and prepositions as well as nouns. When three-word utterances are being used with comfort and regularity an analysis of spontaneous speech will show what types of construction are being developed. This will give a basis for measurement of growth.

Input by the student

This now aims at strengthening the links between statements in order to move on to connected narrative.

Pictures are now useful particularly those which allow the child to project himself into the pictured situation.

STUDENT: 'This boy is happy because it is his birthday. He has got four candles on his cake because he is four. He doesn't go to school because he is only four. When he is five he will go to school. When you are four you will have four candles' *or* 'You had four candles when you were four'

then follow by questions designed to elicit such statements as:

> *When I'm five*
> *When I was four*
> *Because he likes cake*
> *Because he's big*

Then encourage listening and retelling stories. If he came to the clinic on a bus tell him about a bus journey and ask him to tell you about his journey: 'Billy went on the bus with his Mummy. They went to the shops. Mummy bought some oranges and when they got home Billy had one for his tea'.

STUDENT: 'Did you go on a bus?'
CHILD: *'Yes'*
'Where did you go?'
CHILD: *'To* (name of student)'
'Yes, you came to see me didn't you. We can have a story about that'

'One day Danny and his Mummy went to the bus stop to catch a bus. They had to wait a long time. But then the bus came and they got on. Mummy gave the busman some money and they went upstairs. They saw a lot of things from the window. When they were near the clinic Mummy rang the bell and the bus stopped. They both got off the bus and walked down the road. Then they were at the clinic and Miss Blank was there. She said "Hallo Danny".'

Use such narrative as a basis for question and answer. Give the child a toy bus and let him show you where he sat. Emphasise different words and constructions, 'stop', 'wait', 'go'. Use these to direct the child and let him use them to direct you, the bus and then himself. This will encourage him to use verbal directives in controlling and organising his behaviour.

As the child's speech progresses try to build the therapy session around a central theme. Use one game or anecdote as a unifying factor. Make use of role play, question and answer and comment to provide linguistic variety and to strengthen the language matrix.

From now on you should be able to measure progress by means of a linguistic profile such as LARSP. If the child is only delayed and not severely handicapped in language you should now be able to rely upon situational material and varied activities to stimulate language growth. Language has become functional.

Major learning problems

The child will move slowly. He may not be able to deduce language forms and content from a normal linguistic environment. Both input and output need to be structured. In your initial and ongoing assessment always record the use the child makes of his limited resources. He may have only one or two words but they may be used appositely and with expression. He may also accompany them by gesture and general expressivity so that their meaning is enhanced. A child like this is functionally more proficient than a child with the same amount of spoken language but without resource in its use.

Basic techniques

Imitation

Nouns: immediate repetition

Verbs: immediate repetition

Memory training

delayed repetition

supply after noun is said

Always ensure that the child has the necessary concept. If he lacks it use the procedure in the previous chapter.

Aim

To exhibit a simple spoken vocabulary which will enable the child to be understood and thus encourage him to use speech for communication.

STUDENT: 'Let's find the car'

'Here's the car'

'You can say it too – car'

CHILD: *'Car'*

'I wonder if there are any more cars. This looks like a car. Oh, what's this?'

CHILD: *'Car'*

'Now the car's going, its going down the road, the car's ...'

CHILD: *'Go'*

'The car's going down the road. Let's find another one. Here's a blue one. Shall we have this blue one or a red one?'

CHILD: *'Blue'*

Now move to Pivot/open class or use other constructions previously described. As these children need a great deal of reinforcement and consolidation, use plenty of sentence-completion training.

STUDENT: 'He is waiting for his ...'   CHILD: *'Mummy'*

'Mummy's gone into the ...'   *'Shop'*

'She's buying some ...'   *'Sweets'*

'Mummy's in the shop buying
sweets. Who's going to eat them?'   *'Me'*

'Mummy is buying sweets for Danny'

Of course the material used must be adapted to the child's circumstances. The object is to extract as much speech as possible from the child. Use the words that are said most readily and clearly to provide anchor points for simple sentences.

Heighten the child's concentration on listening by using your tape-recorded voice or the tape-recorded voice of another person. Use the recording for sentence-completion work and for memory training.

TAPE-RECORDED VOICE: 'Hallo Danny.   I am the postman. I am going to bring you a letter.   I will drop it through your letter box.   Listen.   Here it comes.   Plop'

STUDENT: 'Who was that?'
'What did he say?' etc.

If the child cannot answer play the tape again. Tell him what the man is going to say.

Now let the child make a record or record him responding to you. Play it back and ask him who is speaking and what was said.

No matter what the nature or degree of the speech delay, make use of what the child offers spontaneously. Respond to his offering at the same level as you conduct the rest of the session.

CHILD: *'Mine'*
STUDENT: 'Oh, what have you got there. May I see?'

CHILD: *'Mine'*
'You've got a new coat. How lovely. Did Mummy buy it for you?'
CHILD: *'Yes'*

Or

STUDENT: 'Who bought that for you?'

CHILD: *'Mummy'*
'Where did she buy it?'
CHILD: *'Shop'*
'Did you go with her?'

Use the incident to provide a basis for a short anecdote as previously described. Remember that making use of the child's spontaneous speech does not mean that the student loses control of the session. If the child is constantly interjecting his own observations you will have to judge whether:

he needs attention training procedures (see Chapter 5);

he is trying to distract you away from the task in hand to something more attractive. If so you must decide whether or not this is justified;

you have not found the appropriate level to engage his interest. Ask yourself whether you are pitching your demands too low or too high.

Further memory training
Check that the child has the necessary level of inhibition and listening ability by asking him to:

'Put your brick in the box when I say – GO'

'Hold it in your hand until I say – GO'

'You have to keep listening because soon I am going to say – GO'

Then proceed to teach a new word:

'We are going to learn a new word. It is cooking. This is what Mummy does when she gets your dinner. She is COOKING the dinner. Here's the picture of Billy's Mummy cooking. Can you say "cooking"? Good. Now listen while I tell you a story.'

'One day Danny was playing outside with his friend Billy. They smelled a lovely smell coming from the house (sniff appreciatively). Billy said, "What's that smell?" Danny said, "My Mummy's cooking the dinner. Let's guess what it is." '

(Ask the child to guess.)

'Then they went inside to see who was right. Danny said, "What are you cooking?" and Mummy said, "I'm cooking a pie." '

Ask the child to repeat the word 'cooking'. Ask his mother to use the word at home and encourage him to use it also.

Never assume that a child knows a word because he has said it once. If it were as simple as that he would have learned it by himself in the first place.

Ask him to:

whisper   sub-vocalise   'lock it up in your head'

Above all see that opportunities are created for use.

No one unit of language is useful by itself. Always make use of appropriate intonation and stress to encourage interest and give extra cues for learning. As soon as any expression is learned make it functional.

These procedures for the child with learning difficulties take us to the point where he may have to be taught verbal constructions. In this way he differs from the language-delayed child who should be able to learn by regular exposure once he has mastered the basic sentence types. Prepare the child with learning difficulties thoroughly by combining his basic vocabulary with intonation which will introduce him to question form as well as statement.

STUDENT (showing a box with items in):   CHILD:
  'Put your hand in and feel one'

  'Is it a big one?'   *'No'*

  'Is it soft?'   *'No'*

  'Is it sticky?'   *'No'*

Play the game with the child and try to induce him to attempt:

  'Soft?' or
  'Sticky?' with rising intonation. Reply appropriately.

Follow by pretend games.

  Child pours tea. *'Want tea?'   'Want milk?'   'Want sugar?'*

Alternative activities and roles to keep question and answer constructions going while you increase length of utterance.

  'Me want biccy. Mummy want biccy?'

When the child has reached this stage allow a couple of months' consolidation before deciding what construction to teach next. This is to allow the child to contribute something of his own if he is able to do so. If he does not take any noticeable steps forward you must decide on the next construction to be taught by:

  reassessing the child's conceptual level,

  studying the literature for the most appropriate language model for this child,

  discussing with his parents how he is performing at home.

With both language-delayed children and those with more severe problems the question of intelligibility is bound to arise. In the early stages of language stimulation and training the material used is closely context-bound. The student is not likely to encounter too many difficulties in deciding on her target. She is aiming at simple syntactical development and within a circumscribed context the child will be intelligible to her. As language output increases, however, judgements will have to be made about articulatory and phonological performance. These areas will be the subject of the next chapter.

If the student is working with children who are showing severe and continuing difficulty in mastering syntax, some form of structured teaching must be devised. This will be the responsibility of the supervising clinician together with the teacher if the child is in school or attending a language unit. The responsibility of the student will be to:

assist in reassessing ... by using LARSP profile or other form of syntax measurement

contribute to the language development programme by finding suitable material for the various stages. It will also be necessary to produce stimulus or teaching material to fill in constructional gaps. It is, therefore, wise to have available:

sets of action pictures *To teach tense*

word lists which contain phonologically simple constructions *To teach vocabulary*

picture showing incidents or activities involving more than one person *To teach comprehension, SVO structures, adverbs, SVOO structures*

Your basic language tools will still be:

Graded questions:
Forced alternatives:

Graded statements:
Using verbal material to hold interest and assist memory

For more functional activities where the child is required to direct you and to give you explicit instructions it is better to use toy material, small objects which may be arranged or handled as directed. This gives the child immediate feedback as to whether his communication has been successful.

Fluency

As language is acquired and spoken language becomes more prolific the child may produce hesitation, repetition, fillers and other non-fluent signs. The student must assess the overall language level to decide whether:

the child is at a developmental stage where such behaviour is appropriate;

the child has inadequate tools for the job he is attempting; this may hinge upon poor vocabulary or inadequate syntax or restricted phonology;

the child is showing speech anxiety ... he lacks confidence in his ability to respond as required;

the child is showing communication anxiety ... his whole situation is too stressful.

Conclusions will be made not only on the basis of your language assessment but outstandingly on the comments of the child's parents and his history. Background help from the literature should be sought using texts on non-fluency and stammering in children.

Management

This will obviously depend on your conclusion.

It is wise to work as calmly and reassuringly as possible whatever the cause.

It is unwise to put too much pressure on the child to speak so concentrate on input.

It is unwise to work on constructions which demand a high degree of precision.

Continue with general stimulation and support and give extra time to parent counselling.

Try to buttress these weak areas by teaching the child the constructions he needs.

In the case of vocabulary and syntax use tactics where you speak and the child identifies. Follow by speaking and letting the child imitate you. Only demand speech from him when you are sure that he has command over the language item.

If the inadequacy seems to be at a phonological level work on discrimination and follow by imitation.

Only ask the child to produce the sound when he can imitate your production.

Spend additional time on recall and delayed repetition to strengthen memory.

In all cases of non-fluency it is useful to use *shadowing* and *modelling*. When using shadowing remember that its success depends upon the child echoing your speech as he hears it but not trying to remember and repeat. So practise with a fellow student until you are well in control of the speed and clarity of your own speech.

When using modelling keep the unit shorter rather than longer so that the child is not overstretched. Use good melodic cadences but keep them simple.

If the child is showing speech or communication anxiety you should not continue to use direct language work.

Speech anxiety
Give the child a brief rest period and ask his parents to see that he is not placed under pressure to speak. Then recommence your language work at the level below the child's standard when the stammering became evident. Consolidate at this level until he is communicating confidently through speech. Give him plenty of chance to listen to speech at the level of his own utterance. Use simple stories which you can record and which the child can replay. Let him join in the telling as he is ready.

Communication anxiety
Investigate the causes as fully as you can. In the meantime place emphasis on communication through play. Seek the help of the educational or clinical psychologist through your supervising speech therapist. Do not abandon the child and his parents but continue to counsel and give relief while considering a future strategy.

CHAPTER 7

The developing sound system: assessment and therapeutic procedures

The child may first present with speech-production difficulties which affect intelligibility or render his speech conspicuous among his peers. The student may also find that delay in the acquisition of normal phonology is one feature of overall language delay (see previous chapter). Decisions as to whether and when speech therapy in the form of direct intervention should be carried out should be based upon thorough assessment. In the case of a child of school age whose speech is described by his mother as 'never easy to understand', 'never clear to people outside the family' or 'he's never pronounced his words clearly (properly)', the decision to intervene may be following the first assessment.

If the accompanying history is one of gradual although slow development it may be preferable to carry out two or three assessments over a period of time to see whether or not the speech is in process of change and if that change is in the direction of normal speech. If so there may be no need for direct treatment.

Assessment

Aims

To establish whether the child can produce the requisite sounds and distinguish them from others

Procedures

oral examination
imitation CV
articulation test
sound discrimination test

To establish whether the child can control his production of the sounds sufficiently to combine them with others

didochokinetic rate
sound sequencing CVC CCV CCVC
speech-discrimination test
phonemic assessment (using articulation or deep articulation test)

To establish whether the child is using his sounds systematically

phonological analysis
speech discrimination

In all forms of assessment it is important to include procedures which will show you whether the child can improve his speech or his production of any sound if he is given a model. *Also* try to establish the extent to which he can self-correct. This will show whether or not he is aware of the adult target and the extent to which he can make use of it. These two factors are very important when estimating prognosis and response to therapy.

The student will find that an experienced clinician will probably start by obtaining a sample of spontaneous speech and will then select from the tools of assessment according to her initial impression of what the problem is. The student should carry out all three procedures, detailed above, until sufficiently experienced to decide between articulation testing and phonological analysis. Never omit the oral examination. This is particularly important if the child is producing sounds which are atypical. Focus of assessment must be upon his articulatory equipment *and his hearing*. However, we are assuming that the student will seek information on the state of the hearing whatever the linguistic features may be.

Articulatory equipment

Questions to be answered
Does the child have the necessary points of contact?

Can he manage the necessary placements?

Can he perform the movements accurately and at speed?

Does he have normal tongue action in speech and nonspeech activities?

Articulation tests

A standardised test appropriate to the child's age should show you whether his phonetic inventory is suitable in range and manner of sound production. Before you embark on such a test prepare the child and the working area. The accuracy of the test will depend upon whether the child responds to all the items. As most such tests use picture stimuli decide whether:

You will let the child turn over the page and/or hold the material	This can hold the child's interest and maintain his co-operation but it can also be very slow and allow other distractions to creep in (e.g. stacking and shuffling cards or turning over two pages at once)
You will control all the material yourself	This keeps the control firmly in your hands but can thereby turn the child into too passive an agent

Also decide whether you are going to encourage conversation between items or forge firmly ahead. A little comment or conversation is more relaxing for you both and allows you to hear more of the child's speech. But too much conversation will defeat the object of the exercise by causing confusion and interference. If you are doubtful whether you can control the child it is wisest to keep comments to a minimum.

Record all speech samples and assessments on the tape recorder as well as graphically. Listen and check your written data. Note whether the recorded speech of the child is less intelligible than he was in the flesh. This will give you some idea of his ability as a total communicator.

Be thorough. Do not use the articulation test simply as a word list. Study the accompanying manual after as well as before administration and make sure that your sample yields you all possible information. Check the results of the articulation test against the results of hearing and oral examinations.

Do the findings agree? If not what questions remain to be answered. For example, have you recorded a number of weak plosives and nasal vowels? If so you must examine:

breath direction
palato-pharyngeal sphincter competence

Are there any overall trends that suggest limited movement? For example, if all front lingual sounds are made with the body of the tongue or the blade, you should re-examine:

tongue action
tongue-tip sensitivity

What is the degree of constancy in the sound production? Remember a constant performance suggests that the child is limited but is organised within his limits. Ask yourself what is imposing the limit:

structural malformation?
developmental immaturity?

If he is inconsistent are the variations:

between normal and abnormal productions?
between immature and very immature productions?

Are the same sounds sometimes present and sometimes not?
How does phonetic context influence production?
What hypothesis can be posed?

Is the child experimenting upon a basis of poor discrimination?
Is he developing towards normal speech (but perhaps un-willingly)?
Is he able to monitor his production?

Phonological analysis

This is carried out to show whether the child's phonetic inventory is being used systematically. If it follows the articulatory assessments listed it should help to formulate the hypothesis.

If the analysis is carried out as the primary procedure it should reveal whether the child's speech is rule governed and if so what are the rules which govern it. How firmly established are these rules?

Data collection

Methods of collecting speech data are discussed in the literature. When your purpose is to carry out a phonological analysis your sample may be more restricted than for grammatical analysis as there is less possible variation. But it is important that you gain a comprehensive sample. Record the child talking with his mother while they are playing. Also record picture description and sentence completion. The last two activities will give you some control over the sounds which are being produced. Tell a story and ask for it to be told back. If the child says little you will need to keep the full corpus of speech for your analysis. If he says a great deal you should try to direct activities so that your tape recording covers a range of contexts. You can then make your analysis from selected tapes.

However, you should also include material which is clearly stuctured so that you are in no doubt as to the target word. A sensible procedure would be:

Naming   STUDENT: *'What is this?'*   CHILD: *'Horse'*

Repetition *'Please say* – *"this old horse is having a drink from the stream"'*

Elicited comment *'What do you think he has been doing?'*

You should try to keep a good supply of pictures of objects and animals so that you can fall back on naming to test the nature of the child's rule, for example:

The child says *'dod'* for *'dog'*

to find whether the sound is present when not influenced by assimilation	a picture of a guy or a sign saying *'go'* a picture of an egg
to establish the influences operating on the sound	a picture of a pig a picture of a log a picture of a Bingo game a picture of a kangaroo

It is obviously simpler to take advantage of procedures already worked out by other people. But try to probe for yourself so that you gain confidence and understanding of what influences a child's production and, therefore, what are the correct and most helpful remedial procedures.

Your phonological analysis should also indicate other trends than phonemic ones. Does the whole pattern show *open syllable?* If so does this tie up with other information, for example, poor short-term auditory memory? What is the next step?

Is the phonological disability strongly influenced by:

coalescence
reduplication
assimilation?

How systematic is the child's speech?

How idiosyncratic is it?

Does it appear to be dominated by one or two abnormally produced sounds which are influencing others?

If so, are these related to structural, motor, auditory deficiencies?

If your examination shows that sounds are produced normally in some words but not in others be sure that the child's parents understand why this is happening. Be prepared to give simple (but not inaccurate) information on how sounds are made and how they influence each other. Ask the child's parents to write down words in which they noticed that certain debatable sounds were said correctly.

Finally try to make some estimate of the discrepancy between phonology and syntax (if present) and the relationship of this mismatch to intelligibility.

Planning and intervention

The result of your assessment will lead to one of many possible conclusions.

No real discrepancy between phonology and syntax.
Development of both is delayed with immature constructions being used.

Treatment Language stimulation, syntactical development

Some discrepancy in that the phonological system is not expanding quickly enough to keep up with developing syntax.

Treatment Speech discrimination, imitation

The phonological system is very restricted and no exploration by the child is evident. He is not attempting to experiment further.

Treatment Auditory discrimination, teaching of distinctive features and establishment of contrasts

The phonology is affected by abnormal production of some sounds; this may be associated with tongue thrusting in which case the practicability of retraining must be considered.

Treatment Sound production using phonetic placement

Articulation is affected by impairment of motor planning or execution; or of auditory impairment or processing.

Treatment Increase mobility and accuracy of articulation, increase speed and range of movement, imitation training, compensatory cueing to assist audition

Articulation is deviant because of structural abnormalities.

Treatment Refer for advice re prosthesis, or compensatory training using principles of acoustic phonetics

All treatment measures are likely to include some aspects of auditory training and/or speech sound production.

Other information

At the conclusion of your assessment you may still be in some doubt as to the exact nature of the child's problem. If so go back over your case history as suggested in Chapter 2. Pay particular attention this time to the child's speech environment.

Who has been the main speech model for the child? If, as is usual, it has been the mother, make an informal assessment of her speech with regard to clarity; rate; vitality; dialect and accent.

If the child has spent a great deal of time with relatives or child minders try to ascertain the status of their speech and hearing.

The number of children in the family, their relative ages and whether the child is a twin or singleton will all affect the nature of the speech environment.

If considerable inconsistencies exist between the clinical and home models, and if there are also inconsistencies at home, they will militate against the success of your auditory training and prevent sounds being stabilised. So before embarking on a course of therapy try to achieve some consistency in the model that the child is offered.

Working with the speech sound system

The distinction between phonology and phonetics is an important one for the clinician. Disorders in a child's speech sound system may result from phonological or phonetic factors or a combination of both. The previous section of this chapter has emphasised the need to obtain a representative sample of the child's speech and your analysis of this sample should provide sufficient information for you to decide why the child is prevented from using a speech sound system suitable for his age. The treatment procedures you choose will depend on this decision.

Guidelines for intervention will come from your knowledge of phonetics, phonological theory and the phonological processes which occur in child speech. The selection of treatment procedures will depend on the theoretical assumptions that are being made but must also include any underlying difficulties presented by the child which may be contributing to the overall problem.

Once a careful and thorough analysis of the child's individual speech patterns has been made you will have to weigh up the presenting evidence and make a judgement on the exact focus of your intervention and the therapeutic strategies you may employ. The solution may not be an easy one and the treatment programme will have to be individually designed to take into account the specific requirements of the child concerned. You are advised to discuss the treatment rationale and procedures for a particular child with your supervising clinician or tutor.

The starting point of any treatment programme designed to help an individual child develop or change his own production will depend upon what the child has to achieve in order for him to do this. To bring about the change required you may need to get into the child's system at one of the levels represented in Figure 4.

Figure 4. Access to the child's speech sound system

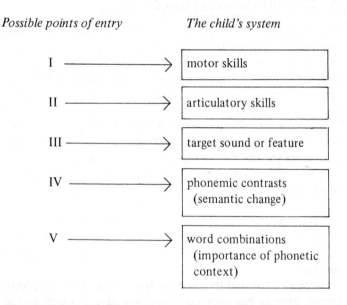

Possible points of entry   *The child's system*

I ⟶ motor skills

II ⟶ articulatory skills

III ⟶ target sound or feature

IV ⟶ phonemic contrasts (semantic change)

V ⟶ word combinations (importance of phonetic context)

If the child has the target sound or feature in his phonemic inventory the treatment programme may begin at level four in the figure above. The aim is to help the child realise the phonemic contrasts of English and achieve these in his own production. Intervention is directed towards changing the child's disordered *patterns* of speech. If, however, the target sound or feature is not present in the child's phonemic inventory, treatment may have to start at one of the earlier levels. It may be necessary to extend the range of sounds available to the child before phonemic contrasts can be introduced. The child must be able to produce the target sound or feature before it can be incorporated into his phonological system. You may have to include specific procedures in your programme to help the child achieve this.

It is unlikely that a treatment programme designed for one child will transfer to another. Once you have decided on the possible starting point for your intervention you must structure your treatment programme around the changes that have to be achieved by the child concerned.

In the following section of this chapter a number of general therapeutic procedures are introduced and you will find many more discussed in your recommended texts. Treatment can rarely be prescriptive and the selection of appropriate procedures and techniques, the exact nature of intervention and the content of any programme will vary for each child.

Some general therapeutic procedures

Inducing change and structuring context

Try to elicit any change in the child's speech sound system by using straightforward *imitation techniques* first.

Whenever possible induce the change in a *meaningful context* where the communicative value of the change is stressed. This is particularly important if your therapy is directed towards the organisation of contrastive elements in the child's phonological system. The use of word pairs (minimal pairs or minimal sets) is one way of doing this. It is important to check that the child can understand and discriminate the words you have selected and is aware of what he is aiming for. A simple story might be used to encompass these activities.

Example

THERAPIST: 'This man lives in a castle and has lots of money. He is very rich. This old lady with the black cat and the broomstick is a witch.

Can you show me the one who is rich ...

Now show me the witch.

Listen, I'm going to tell you a story about a rich man and a witch ...'

(Tell simple story using the paired words several times.)

'Can you hear I am using two different sounds when I say rich and witch. Let's see if you can copy me and then you can help tell the story.'

In most programmes you will have to include procedures to encourage and motivate the child to *change his own production*. Some children are sensitive to the adult model and try to match it, whilst others do little to modify their own speech patterns despite satisfactory listening and discrimination skills. You should try to include perception/production links at strategic points in your programme. Use the child's good perceptual abilities to focus attention on the changes he has to make in his own production in order to be understood. Various techniques can be used to achieve this. The following examples illustrate a few of these:

Example

THERAPIST: (offering a choice of small toys)
'Which one would you like?'
CHILD: *'Shoe'* [tu]
'Two? Do you mean another one like   Requesting
that?'   clarification
(pointing to a toy already on the table)
   'No ... a shoe' [sju]
(accepting the child's attempt at
change)   Providing a
'Oh a shoe'   model

(nods)
'Well I have a red shoe and a black
shoe in my box
Which one would you like?'
  'A red shoe' [sju]
'Say red *shoe*'
  'Red shoe' [ʃu]
'Good, you said that very well'

Providing
additional
models

Requesting imitation

Informing child
that his attempt
was successful

Example

THERAPIST: 'Now which piece
would you like for the puzzle?'
CHILD: [gɛə]
'A bear?'   Check question
  (*reaches out, but the piece is
  withheld*)
'If you want it you must say   Requesting imitation
bear'   from model
  'Bear' [bɛə]
(gives the child the first piece and
offers another)
'And here's another ......'
  'Bear' [gɛə]
(withholds the piece and looks   non-spoken
at the child in mock disapproval)   signal for
                                         change

(grinning) 'Bear' [bɛə]

Consideration must be given to the influence of *phonetic
context* on the child's production of sound contrasts. For example, a child may be able to realise /k/ in words such as *car* and
key before he can achieve this in *coat* and *cat*. The phonetic

context may have to be carefully structured in the early stages of a programme but the aim should be to help the child to achieve his target in various phonetic contexts. You may have to anticipate the possible influence of phonetic context on an individual child's production when selecting words and word combinations.

The use of specific therapeutic techniques

Some additional therapeutic procedures may have to be included in your overall therapy programme if the child concerned cannot achieve change through discrimination and imitation of the adult model. He may require specific help to produce the targets needed to develop or expand his phonological system. Try to work out from your assessment what factors may be imposing the limitation on the child and adapt your therapy programme accordingly.

Facilitating movement

You may have to include work on *facilitating movements* if your assessment shows that the child's overall system is constrained by limited mobility of the speech organs or if the child is having difficulty in controlling accurate, differentiated movements of the tongue or lips at speed.

If this is the case, you may have to begin by increasing the child's oral sensitivity and help him achieve the required articulatory gesture by manipulating the tongue, lips or jaw.

Never insist on a particular movement if by doing so you distort the child's whole system or cause exaggerated production.

Your short-term aim may be to increase the child's range and speed of movements but remember that your long-term aim is to improve the child's communicative function. Once you have achieved some differentiated and controlled movements you should try to help the child use these to produce contrastive phonemes at a word level.

Assisting placement

If your assessment shows that a particular articulatory placement is *absent* from the child's system you may have to help him acquire the additional placement so that new articulatory gestures become available to him. Again you may need to increase the child's oral sensitivity and elicit the new placement by stimulating the position or contact required by the tongue or lips. You may be able to achieve the placement by using visual cues and demonstrations or by assisting with a tongue blade or physical prompts.

Once the child can make the target sounds at the new placement help him to incorporate the additional phonemic contrasts into his phonological system.

Eliciting sounds

Your assessment may show that the child's system is affected by an atypical production of a particular phoneme. The child may be using the deviant sound contrastively within his system so that his speech is conspicuous rather than unintelligible. You may have to *elicit the target sound* if the child is unable to produce it by other means.

You will find various suggestions for eliciting consonants in the classic texts on speech pathology. Before attempting to elicit the target sound work out how the child's deviant production differs from the target and whether you need to do any preliminary work on helping the child inhibit a faulty movement or posture.

Example

> The child may first have to learn to inhibit lower lip involvement and compensatory jaw movement before he can achieve the tongue-tip activity required for the production of /r/

Elicitation techniques should be based on your knowledge of phonetics and you may be able to use a consonant or vowel which is already in the child's system as a starting point.

Example

> Using a slow release of the tongue tip from /t/ with accentu-
> ated aspiration to lead to /s/

Rehearsing

Some children may need time to *rehearse* a newly acquired skill
in order to gain sufficient control over it. If this is the case you
may have to include practice initially in a non-linguistic context
until the child can produce the target sound smoothly, at speed
and combine it with other sounds. Once the child has gained
control, direct your therapy to the word and phrase level as soon
as possible.

Listening training

You may have to include specific *listening training* at certain
points in your programme, especially if your assessment has
shown that the child has difficulties with speech discrimination.
The aim of auditory discrimination tasks is to help the child
notice contrasts to prepare him for the changes he has to make
in his own production. Remember that listening for meaning is
very different from listening to detail. The first is a much more
fundamental part of communication and you may have to begin
training at the word level before the phoneme level.

Children with specific auditory perceptual problems may need
a greater emphasis on this aspect of therapy but the procedures
involved are beyond the scope of this introductory chapter.

The final consideration in any programme is the carry-over
into conversational speech. Once the child has demonstrated
consistent control over the desired target in a structured context,
emphasis must be placed on encouraging the child to incorporate
the change into his spontaneous utterances. It is important to
involve the adults most closely concerned with the child from
the start of your treatment. The adults have to serve in a recep-
tive capacity and monitor the child. They will probably learn

best from watching the clinician at work and noting the strategies the therapist employs to bring about change in the child's production. Try to keep the adults concerned in touch with what you are doing, why you are doing it and inform them about their role. The parents should be encouraged to stimulate verbal activity and they should be guided as to whether a particular production should be reinforced or not.

CHAPTER 8

Language use: alternative treatment strategies

As we set out to teach language, we are in danger of misdirecting our efforts if we restrict our aims to helping the child produce good language forms (syntax, phonology and intonation). The acquisition of appropriate language forms is of course important, and such skills must be made available to children. However, good language forms are only necessary to serve a purpose, which is to allow the child to communicate effectively in his environment. Language serves social purposes: it is used to exchange meanings, to develop ideas and to facilitate social interaction. Children learn language because they have things to say, and because they wish to talk to people who are socially important to them.

Language can also be used privately, to direct oneself and one's own behaviour. This second purpose of language is intra- rather than inter-personal, and is not directly social in its intention. This type of language also shows development, but it is the social use of language which will be the main focus of this chapter.

Therapists must aim to teach the child good language skills which are used to serve valid social purposes. This aim means that therapists enter into social interactions with two separate and somewhat contradictory purposes in mind. The first is to exchange meanings with the child, to receive and respond to his ideas and to contribute her own. The second, perhaps conflicting, aim is to influence the child's language productions, and therapists interact with children in order to do this. This second purpose distinguishes speech therapists and language teachers from most other conversationalists, who may wish to influence their partners' actions, but who have no wish to interfere with their speech styles. Parents of normally developing children, who might be expected to resemble language therapists in this respect, appear to be concerned with the accurate interpretation of meanings and only rarely with the quality of speech productions. Therapists must take both aspects of their communicative behaviour into account.

In order to achieve these dissonant purposes, speech therapists must develop language intervention strategies which impinge upon children's language output while continuing to promote communication. It is necessary to develop techniques which achieve both aims at once. To concentrate exclusively on language forms without considering language use is to take the risk that new skills will be acquired and used in structured practice sessions in the speech clinic, but will be dropped when the child enters a 'real' conversation. This difficulty in 'carrying over' newly acquired skills to real-life situations has long been recognised in therapy, and is a problem which absorbs much of the clinician's time and energy.

This chapter outlines some techniques which serve the therapist's aim of improving language forms and use, but which interfere minimally with communication and the exchange of meanings.

Techniques

Use of language forms — syntax and phonology

Once the syntactic or phonological feature has been selected for carry-over training, it is useful simply to increase the number of times the child hears it. Using the feature frequently in conversation will tend to encourage the child to do the same.

It appears that children can use the adult's speech form as a model from which to extract relevant features. Use of modelling has already been discussed (Chapter 5) and further examples will be given here.

Examples

1. Expansion

Here the child's own utterance is repeated, with the addition of the selected feature omitted by the child. This will often encourage the child to re-echo his utterance, incorporating the new feature. Thus,

THERAPIST: 'How many children are there?'
CHILD: *'One boy two girl'*
'A boy and two girls'
CHILD: *'Yes, two girls'*

Extra information can be given along with the expansion, to take the meaning further and so encompass both of the therapist's aims.

2. 'Check' questions

The 'check' question is prompted by the genuine communication need to be sure that the child's meaning has been correctly received. 'Check' or 'echo' questions once again give the child a model of how he could have phrased his utterance, and how the new feature is used.

THERAPIST: 'What's he called?'
CHILD: *'That's the sheriff'* ['tɛwɪ]
'Sheriff?' ['ʃɛɹɪf]
CHILD: *'Yea, the sheriff'* ['ʃɛwɪ] = + /ʃ/

3. Forced alternative questions

The use of forced alternative questions obliges the child to produce the required feature to clarify his meaning.

CHILD: *'It a box'*
THERAPIST: 'It *is* a box, or it's *not* a box?'
'It is a box'

Therefore, these three modelling techniques can be used by the therapist in conversation with the child, to improve the child's use of a syntactic or phonological feature while at the same time allowing him to develop his meanings. Modelling techniques are taken from naturally occurring conversational devices, and are therefore seldom out of place in 'real' social situations.

Use of language — interesting communication

For many children, our aim is to encourage them to use the language skills they already possess in an appropriate and flexible manner. Children who possess good language skills, but do not use them, have just as great a language difficulty as children with syntactic and phonological problems. We must therefore develop intervention strategies to encourage aspects of language use.

When doing this, the guiding principle is to follow the child's lead; to accept his initiations, to keep the conversation going and to develop it. The opposite strategy, of imposing too great a control on the discourse, and giving the impression that there is a 'right answer' which must be arrived at by the child, is a strategy which prevents interesting communication taking place (at least from the child's point of view) and may dampen the child's enthusiasm for conversation.

The techniques employed to encourage language use will vary with the child's ability to code his meanings and with the structural complexity of his utterance. It is nonetheless possible to identify techniques of general applicability. Four areas of language use will therefore be considered: *topics, questions, repair* and *context.*

Topics

Children will use language if there is a meaning which they want to convey. What constitutes an interesting topic will vary from child to child. Some children will choose to communicate about novel, dramatic events, others are frightened of and resist change, and do not wish to communicate about over-exciting events. Information about individual preferences can be obtained by observing the circumstances in which a child chooses to communicate.

Young language-learning children normally comment on obvious features of the environment, and do not give 'new' information unless it is specifically requested, and this type of language may be expected from developmentally young children. As this may be a feature which is more closely related to cognitive rather than linguistic development, a child with cognitive development in advance of language development would not be expected to comment exclusively on features present in the communication environment, but to transcend them. An example of the first type of comment is:

CHILD: *'Go there'*
THERAPIST: 'Doesn't. It goes there. Turn it round. Good. Very good indeed.'
CHILD: *'I've won'*
'You've won, yes'
CHILD: *'That the clock'*
'You've got the clock' etc.

The example of the second type of comment is taken from the speech of an older language-disordered child:

THERAPIST: 'Can you *tell* us the story about King Wenceslas?'
CHILD: *'Beverley walked on table. Sit chair'* etc.

Once again, it is necessary to observe the child's communication level and his level of development to assess which type of comment can be encouraged.

Certain conversation topics appear to interest most children. Planning and organising special events, and later discussing them, can elicit a great deal of language. One of the most fascinating topics, to most adults as well as children, is *ourselves*: our own experiences, our homes and families, what our pets do and eat, and how we feel about our friends. In the following example, a rather taciturn child responded to a lucky question from the therapist, asking if she had any pets.

Example

THERAPIST: 'Four? Well, I can think of a dog and a cat, is that two of them? And what else have you got?'
CHILD: *'A horse'*
'A horse?'
CHILD: *'And a pony'*
'Pony? Have you? Do you ride on them?'
CHILD: *'Yes'*
'Both of them, or just the pony?'
CHILD: *'My mum rides horse, I pony'*

However, it is often sensible to find out about a child's interests in the hope that likely topics will be suggested.

Photographs of children and their friends and relations can also be used to elicit conversation and comment, and the advent of the polaroid camera has made possible the immediate recording of events. Many children have favourite television programmes and are willing to tell you the 'story'. This topic can elicit examples of narrative speech, and sometimes discussion of the motivation of TV characters, and can lead to interesting conversations.

Many therapists will choose a conversation topic about which they have some knowledge, in order to predict to some extent what the child may say, to help with intelligibility problems and syntactic limitations. This is a sensible strategy, as long as it is not used to cut across a preferred topic chosen by the child. Some controlled deception might be necessary, with the therapist neglecting to reveal all she knows already about a topic, and allowing the child to teach her new tasks.

To extend the notion of *topic*, therapists may have to select the words which are to be taught to children. If so, it is worth noting that certain words are more useful than others. A child who learns to say *'ball'*, *'cup'* and *'spoon'* can demand and comment upon balls, cups and spoons, but nothing else. If, instead of being taught to label specific objects, the child has learned words which could be related to many objects, and situations, he would be in a much better position to influence his environment. Thus, words such as *'more'*, *'that'*, *'me'* and *'no'*, together with *'mummy'* or *'daddy'*, may be likely candidates for much early language teaching. These words are most useful, and therefore likely to be used by children, and will make a wide variety of topics available to the child.

Questions

Conversations between language-disordered children and adults are characterised by the large number of questions asked by the adult. This is such a noticeable feature that the first technique to consider is whether a straightforward decrease in the number of adult questions to the child would show benefits by allowing the child space to develop the discourse in a way interesting to him.

Many adult questions are prompted by different communication needs. One need is to check that the adult has correctly decoded the child's meaning before responding to that meaning. These 'check' questions have already been discussed when considering ways of changing language forms, and are prompted by a genuine communication purpose, based on the need accurately to exchange meanings in conversation. 'Check' questions may be a necessary part of the negotiation of meaning, especially when conversing with a child with language difficulties. They must therefore be retained to serve this purpose. They are less useful as a mere habitual response to allow the therapist time to think.

Another set of questions is designed to further the discourse, where the child is asked for 'new' information, which is unknown to the therapist. For example:

THERAPIST: 'Is there a new park?'
CHILD: *'Yes'*
'Where?'
CHILD: *'Cross the road, our house'*

Such questions are also prompted by communication demands, and do therefore encourage the child to use language.

A third communication need which appears to prompt questions is the adult's need to get the child to say *something*, no matter what. This often happens when the child does not obey turn-taking rules, and the adult feels that only direct questions will elicit speech. Such questions may not serve useful communication purposes, and may extend a 'conversation' where neither partner has a great interest in the topic.

Such 'conversations' have got little to do with sharing meanings. In most instances the adult questioner is firmly controlling the direction of the discourse, and is asking a set of questions for which there is a correct answer, already known to the adult, which must be arrived at by the child. For example:

THERAPIST: 'What's this?'
CHILD: *'A brick'*
'Yes, what colour is it?'
CHILD: *'Blue'*
'No, it's red. How many bricks are there?'
CHILD: *'Four'*
'No, there's five'
etc.

In this sort of conversation, no meanings are exchanged. The adult has already determined the meaning, and is refusing to share it with the child. Such a questioning style is useful for a limited number of didactic purposes, but it is not likely to develop creative use of language. One reason for its limitations is the fact that closed questions of this type require only one-word answers, and therefore there is little chance of developing the form or the content of the discourse.

This question style is one which is very likely to arise when picture description is used as the topic of conversation. Pictures impose certain constraints upon discourse, and perhaps encourage the inexperienced student to produce a number of 'wh–' questions ('What's this?', 'What's he doing?' etc.) without being able to develop the discourse. For such reasons, it is in many cases unwise to make picture description the main basis of language teaching.

When pictures are used, a more general question, such as 'What can we see?', will allow the child an opportunity to place his own meaning on the item. If he produces a string of stereotyped phrases, (*'The boy is walking', 'The girl is sitting'* etc.) which many children have been trained to do, it might be possible to redirect the child's attention to the theme of the picture, and perhaps to ask *why* certain things are occurring, in the child's opinion.

The above discussion assumes that your aim is to encourage the use of language, and to raise the frequency and quality of response. There are times, however, when we wish to *decrease* the amount of irrelevant, off-topic, perhaps stereotyped speech produced by the child. For these occasions, a number of 'conversation stopper' questions, which give control to the adult, might be useful techniques to apply.

Repair

Repair techniques are employed if communication breaks down and is an attempt by both parties to re-establish a meaningful exchange. Typically, one partner (A) makes a statement, and his partner (B) misunderstands his meaning or intention. B may not realise that he has misunderstood, in which case he makes a *non-sequitur* response. A may therefore realise that there has been a misapprehension. Partner A may then signal that partner B has misunderstood, and try to amend the communication failure. Alternatively, partner B may realise that he has not understood A, in which case he will either signal the fact to A, or adopt a 'wait and see' policy, to see if A's later statements clear up the muddle. If this does not happen, partner B will request clarification. Figure 5 represents the process diagramatically.

Figure 5

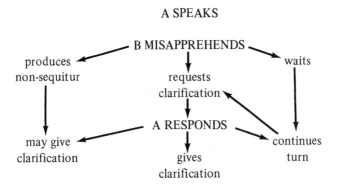

There are several ways in which clarification can be requested, and these in turn control the clarification offered. One type of clarification request, the recapitulatory check question has already been discussed. However, the key feature of successful repair to be discussed here occurs *before* clarification is offered, when one conversational partner realises that a misapprehension has taken place, and signals the fact to the other partner. This is usually done close to the source of the difficulty, so that the misapprehension is cleared up quickly and communication can continue.

Many children with language difficulties, almost by definition, suffer a great deal of communication failure. However, they are not always proficient at dealing with the problem and communication repair is a skill which may have to be taught.

Children need to learn both halves of the repair process – how to signal that they have not understood, and how to improve their own message after it has been misunderstood by another.

Due to comprehension problems, many children do find adult speech difficult to decode. However, it is rare for them to ask for clarification, preferring to adopt a 'wait and see' strategy. This is not particularly helpful, since the misapprehension is not signalled and cannot be cleared up. The following example, taken from a conversation with a mentally handicapped adult and his mother, shows the sort of difficulty which can arise if a misapprehension is not sorted out in time.

Example

THERAPIST: 'And what do you do at lunch time? When it's your recreation time?'
ADULT: ['ɹɛkn] *'time'*
THERAPIST: 'What do you do then?'
(four-second pause)
MOTHER: (whispers) 'What do you do after you've had your dinner?'
ADULT: *'Me dinner!'*
THERAPIST: 'After dinner'
MOTHER: 'After dinner'
ADULT: *'After dinner'*

Had this adult indicated that he had not understood the therapist's original question, much confusion could have been avoided.

It is not surprising that children often refrain from asking adults to clarify their communications. Adults assume the dominant role in many interactions, and it may seem almost rude to ask them to clarify their meanings. Furthermore, many children are aware that they have language problems, and accept much of the responsibility for communication failure. They are therefore unlikely to ask another to repair communication breakdown.

For these reasons, it is often necessary to teach a child specific strategies for signalling communication distress. A general 'all purpose' query such as *'Sorry?'* or *'Pardon?'* are among the most useful forms, and are likely to elicit a repetition of the original statement. Alternatively, the child can say *'I don't understand'*, which is likely to encourage the other to reformulate his message entirely. The following example shows how this can operate.

Child A: 'Where you live?'
Child B: 'Pardon?'
Child A: 'Where you live?'
Child B: 'Longton Street'
Child A: 'Huh?'
Child B: 'Longton Street'
Child A: 'Hm'

It is often necessary to tell the child what to say when he does not understand, and to give him permission to do this in conversation. This is an extremely important use of language skill, and an area in which straightforward training can pay dividends.

Children must also learn to respond to adult requests for clarification of their messages, and student therapists must know which type of request will help the child to do this. One form of the clarification request, the check question mentioned above, provides the child with a useful model of how he might have produced his utterance. Another form of the request for clarification specifies which part of the utterance is causing the problem, and encourages the child to repeat that part, as in the following example.

Example

CHILD: *'Zebra'*
ADULT: 'A what?'
CHILD: *'Like a zebra crossing'*
'Like a what?'
CHILD: *'A zebra'*

This form of request tells the child more about the specific problem, but gives him no model to help him to change.

The third type of clarification request seems to be used when adults cannot make a guess about what a child might have said, and uses an all-purpose form such as 'What?' or 'Pardon?' This signals to the child that he must revise his message, but gives no clue as to how it should be done. It may therefore be a less useful form than either of the other two.

Context

The context in which communication occurs is important, because it forms part of the 'given' information in the situation to which conversational partners may orientate. It is possible to manipulate the communication context to influence the language produced, and of course the language used must have a reciprocal relationship with the context. Certain contextual variations place obligations upon conversational partners to use more or less explicit language, and can therefore be used as language facilitation techniques.

Context has been manipulated artificially in some instances, by using, for example, the 'referential' communication situation, where language partners are separated from each other by a screen, and must use particularly exact language to direct the other's unseen movements. This has obvious uses for encouraging certain types of language, and is an example of manipulating the environment to make particular uses of language more likely to occur.

As we are searching for intervention techniques which are as natural as possible, it is worth considering that many children's games provide a context which resembles the referential situation as an integral part of the game. Adaptations of Happy Families, Picture Lotto and Funny Men Snap can be played like this, where the child has to make an exact description of the card he is holding, unseen by other players, before another child can claim it as matching his own. The exact use of language can therefore be elicited in a somewhat more familiar context.

Certain other manipulations of context can be used to encourage children to speak. An adult who says firmly 'I'm going to put all the cards away in the box now' and *leaves one out*, is highly likely to have her mistake pointed out by a child. Similarly, searching for something with a great deal of comment when it is within the child's vision, but not in yours, is likely to elicit comment. There are many situations which can be manipulated to allow, and indeed to oblige, the child to use his language skills.

There is one further aspect of language use which can be considered under the heading of context, and that is the effect which the child's use of language is allowed to have on his environment. We act through speech, and use language to manipulate others in our environment to achieve specific ends. The amount of control we have over our environment is of course subject to a number of checks, but for language to have a purpose, at least some of the child's legitimate demands upon his environment should be heeded.

There is a danger, especially with handicapped children, that we remove this force from language. We ask a question, such as 'What programme do you want to watch?', but do not heed the answer, saying 'No, we'll watch the other one instead', preferring to 'know better' than the child. To receive this response on occasion is part of the regular give and take of human interactions: but if all our requests meet this sort of response, language ceases to be effective, and may cease to be used.

We must, therefore, allow language-disordered children to mean what they say, to allow them to use language to exercise choice, and to influence their surroundings using speech. Most children have this freedom, and learn to express more explicit meanings by paying attention to the consequences of their speech. If an institutional setting militates against such choice, language for the children concerned may cease to have any meaning.

Principles

When considering how to help the child use language, it is not sufficient to consider the child's language forms, or even the child's present use of language, but to consider the social settings in which the child speaks. As therapists, we are part of that social scheme, and it is just as important to study our language to the child as to study his reciprocal productions. This can be a somewhat dispiriting exercise, but in the end it is an essential one. As we are included among the child's communication partners, we are ideally situated to influence his language use and to teach him to become a skilled communicator.

CHAPTER 9

Working through other people

The practising speech therapist may choose to work in one or all of the following ways:

1. She carries out treatment herself. Although the overall assessment and diagnostic procedures will be shared with other people the speech therapist subsequently decides how the speech change is to be effected and carries this through by personal intervention.

2. The speech therapist defines the problems and asks other people to use their skills to remedy it.

3. She combines her skills with those of other professionals to produce programmes which may then be administered by any one of the professional workers.

4. The speech therapist breaks the task down into a series of sub-tasks and her own skills into a series of sub-skills. She then instructs others in the use of the sub-skills to attack the sub-tasks.

The first category is the classic career role and is most likely to be that which has attracted the student into the profession. It is the category in which the student must become competent and in which she must feel confident. If not she will be unable to make her proper professional contribution.

The second category is that of consultant. Here the speech therapist must be able to appreciate the significance of the com-municative behaviour and suggest the person whose skills or attributes may best effect the desired change. This judgement is the remit of the experienced clinician. Students may take part in the evaluation and observe the subsequent discussion and recommendations. As their experience increases they may be able to make suggestions as to management.

The third category is responsible for communicative programmes involving those children who have needs additional to speech therapy. Examples can be found in the cerebral-palsied and mentally retarded populations. Clearly defined and co-ordinated programmes are also used in schools or units for the language disordered. Here teachers and psychologists form part of the team. The speech therapy student carrying out her clinical practice in any specialised establishment must acquaint herself very throughly with the method which is being employed. She should not make any changes in her procedure without discussion with all other team members. She is no longer responsible only to her supervising speech therapist but to the team as a whole. Although the contribution of the experienced speech therapist is greater than that of an inexperienced student the latter may contribute very helpfully and may gain professional expertise. It is not desirable, however, that any speech therapy student works in such a team for the major part of her clinical training as she will not gain the experience necessary for professional independence through having to use her individual judgement and having to experiment with a variety of techniques.

The fourth category is that of adviser or guide. Here the speech therapist is asking other people to do something they are not automatically equipped to do. They are being asked to carry out tasks which they would not normally undertake and without knowledge of the whole task which has yielded their particular sub-task. The speech therapist giving the advice must, therefore, have a very clear idea indeed of the nature of the problem, and be able to see how each individual element contributes to the whole. While this would seem to demand a very experienced clinician, students frequently find themselves in this role. They may be asked to show a child's mother how to practise with him or to instruct an aide in the management of an institutionalised child.

It is likely that the student herself is being trained by a mixture of these categories. If she is aware of the training process as it affects herself she may be more quickly able to apply it to others.

Training of the student

She observes the speech therapist and carries out small tasks as required.

She regularly undertakes specific procedures of a routine nature. For example she will assist the child to say words containing a newly acquired sound by giving praise or by insisting on another attempt. Or she may carry out an exercise in auditory discrimination between two phonemes. If the student is attending a clinic on a weekly basis and other students attend on different days this kind of assistance may be all she is required to do. If, however, she is the only student assistant she will progress more rapidly to initiating treatment. She will, therefore, also be able to appraise the effect on a child of having too many people intervening with his speech and appreciate the need for clarity of explanation and consistency in carrying out any practice. She will also appreciate the importance of observation before carrying out any procedure, however small.

In order to move to the next phase the student must have a thorough theoretical grounding. She will then be able:

to suggest appropriate procedures which her supervising clinician will approve. The student then carries out treatment of her own devising through personal intervention. As she becomes experienced she is in fact learning the timing as well as the nature of therapeutic intervention. The more conscious she is of the timing of the individual elements, the more likely she is to achieve success. If she does not become really aware of what she is doing and why, she may achieve sporadic success, but will not be able to rely on her techniques and so she will not be able to share them with others.

Awareness can be cultivated by the same kind of observation which the student therapist has been required to give to others. She must learn to sit slightly outside herself even when most enthusiastically involved in order to assess the effectiveness of her actions and to note the child's response in every particular. Then a careful log book or clinical casebook must be kept to give a full working account of the procedures and their effect. Recording the speech therapy session is invaluable for recapitulatory study.

The speech therapy student may also grow into the role of adviser by being observed during her therapy sessions by parents and others who wish to assist. The questions asked will stimulate the student to think clearly about what she is doing. This kind of observation is different from that of her supervisor but may at first be equally intimidating.

Observation by the supervising clinician

The purpose of this observation is to assist the student to develop as a clinician. The supervisor will note:

the relationship which the student is able to initiate and maintain with the child

the material which has been prepared

the manner in which the material is used

the appropriateness of all the procedures

the timing of the procedures

the readiness of the student to take a lead from the child and to turn it into an appropriate therapeutic activity the duration of the whole session and the way in which it is wound up

whether or not the child appears to have derived benefit

The supervisor will then discuss the session with the student in order to consolidate the good points and see how the weaker ones may be changed. Such discussion will seek to draw upon the theoretical basis of the treatment, the extent to which the student understands the condition and its manifestations in this particular child.

Demonstrations and discussions of this kind are an admirable and essential preparation for the student who is learning to work with parents and others responsible for the child's welfare. She may learn from her own supervision the impression she is making on another person. If it is considered helpful the sessions may be video-taped so that they are available during discussion and for further study.

A student who is asked to conduct treatment in the presence of an observer should, therefore, remind herself that the request would not have been made unless her supervising clinician considered that she was capable of representing speech therapy.

Observation by accompanying parent

The parent is likely to note:

the manner of the student towards the child; whether she likes and accepts the child and, therefore, enables the child to accept therapy

whether the student can control the child without harshness

the usefulness of the session as a whole; whether it has justified the time spent in coming to the clinic

whether the student can make a change in the child's behaviour by clear management and tactics whether the student is resourceful in finding ways of helping the child

whether the child enjoyed the session and will willingly come again.

In subsequent discussion the parent will want to know how the child is getting on and what she can do to help. While the student must take care not to usurp the authority of the speech therapist in charge, she must be ready to discuss the child's speech or language difficulty and explain exactly what she is trying to do. This includes:

the present state of the child's language

the immediate steps to be taken

the way in which general support can be given

the manner in which any specific practice should be carried out.

Practice entered in a book should be clearly written and illustrated and also explained and discussed with parent and child. Suggestions should be made as to how often the practice should be carried out and for how long.

The parent will note whether or not the student appears to understand the parent's position. A young student can appear at a disadvantage unless she makes an effort to appreciate the working life of parents and the demands on their time. Naive assumptions as to the ready availability of time and money will reduce credibility. The student should take care to acquaint herself with the family circumstances or, if she took the initial history, to remind herself of these circumstances.

Parent demonstrations of this nature are a very good preparation for the next stage of work which is to construct programmes for other people to carry out. In the case of such programmes the emphasis is shifted. The student is less concerned about demonstrating the way in which she herself works as in explaining the condition, the way in which it can be altered and the goals and sub-goals involved in the alteration. She is constructing treatment which depends for its success not on her own personality and aptitude but on the abilities of another person.

This is a highly skilled task and cannot be carried out successfully until the student has had a considerable amount of practice with similar cases. Without practical experience to guide judgement there is a danger that programmes will be impracticable for others to use, either because they are too detailed or because they are too cursory.

The student may prepare herself for her role as adviser by careful task analysis. Her clinical casebook will be a major source of reference. Her capabilities as an adviser will be a good indication of clinical growth.

Clinical growth

The speech therapy student is attempting to become proficient in order to enter the profession. Once entered she will contribute to the growth and status of this profession. Clinical practice under supervision must be undertaken in order that the student may be qualified in those techniques which the profession has found to be valuable and with which it is associated. It is also demanded in order that the student may learn how to make use of theory in the devising and implementation of diagnostic and remedial procedures. The student is being given a methodology to carry her through the wide field of communication disorder. She is therefore asked to see herself both as a trainee and as a future contributor. In the first function she must be meticulous and attentive, in the second insightful and exploratory. The clinical setting in which a student is trained may not be that in which she wishes to practice. It will be part of clinical training to learn how to judge the suitability of the setting in relation to the purpose for which it is being used. The relationship of setting and method comprise much of the management of a case.

Students may find it helpful to read Chapters 2, 3 and 4 of *Speech Therapy: Principles and Practice* (Byers Brown, 1981) with regard to speech therapy procedures and the environments in which they are pursued. Increased knowledge and new thinking will suggest new settings for old techniques and will generate new techniques to be employed in the clinic and in the community (see Chapter 4, *Speech Therapy*).

The procedures given in this manual are basic and as such are intended to contribute to straightforward proficiency and simple self-confidence. Once they have been mastered real clinical growth can start. Unless they can be carried out easily and pleasurably real proficiency will be postponed and confidence eroded. The rich clinical rewards of working with young children will therefore prove elusive.

Bibliography

You will have been given references and reading lists to support and supplement your lectures.

The following are recommended to help you with the practical aspects of your clinical work.

Antony, A., Boyle, D., Ingram, T.T.S. and McIsaac, M.W. (1971) *The Edinburgh Articulation Test*. Churchill Livingstone, Edinburgh.

Brimer, M.A. and Dunn, L.M. (1973) *The English Picture Vocabulary Test*. N.F.E.R. Publishing Co., Windsor.

Byers Brown, B. (1981) *Speech Therapy: Principles and Practice*. Churchill Livingstone, Edinburgh.

Carrow, E. (1973) *Test for Auditory Comprehension of Language*. N.F.E.R. Publishing Co., Windsor.

Cooper, J., Moodley, M. and Reynell, J. (1978) *Helping Language Development: A Developmental Programme for Children with Early Language Handicaps*. Edward Arnold, London.

Crystal, D. (1979) *Working with LARSP: Studies in Language Disability and Remediation 1A*. Edward Arnold, London.

Crystal, D., Fletcher, P. and Graham, M. (1976) *The Grammatical Analysis of Language Disability: Studies in Language Disability and Remediation 1*. Edward Arnold, London.

Crystal, D., Fletcher, P. and Graham, M. (1981) *A Language Assessment, Remediation and Screening Procedure (revised)*. University of Reading.

Finnie, N.R. (1974) second edition. *Handling the Young Cerebral Palsied Child at Home*. William Heinemann Medical Books, London.

Frazer, W.I. and Grieve, R. (1981) *Communicating with Normal and Retarded Children*. John Wright & Sons, Bristol.

Gillham, B. (1979) *The First Word Language Programme*. George Allen & Unwin, London.

Goldman, R. and Fristoe, M. (1972) *Test of Articulation*. N.F.E.R. Publishing Co., Windsor.

Gordon, N. and McKinlay, I. (eds) (1980) *Helping Clumsy Children*. Churchill Livingstone, Edinburgh.

Ingram, D. (1976) *Phonological Disability in Children: Studies in Language Disability and Remediation 25*. Edward Arnold, London.

Ingram, D. (1981) *Procedures for the Phonological Analysis of Children's Language*. University Park Press, Baltimore.

Jeffree, D. and McConkey, R. (1976) *Let Me Speak*. Human Horizons Series, Souvenir Press, London.

Jeffree, D.M. and McConkey, R. (1976) *P.I.P. Developmental Charts*. Hodder & Stoughton, Sevenoaks.

Jeffree, D.M., McConkey, R. and Hewson, S. (1977) *Let Me Play*. Human Horizons Series, Souvenir Press, London.

Jeffree, D.M., McConkey, R. and Hewson, S. (1977) *Teaching the Handicapped Child*. Human Horizons Series, Souvenir Press, London.

Jeffree, D.M. and Skeffington, M. (1980) *Let Me Read*. Human Horizons Series, Souvenir Press, London.

Knowles, W. and Masidlover, M. (1982) *Derbyshire Language Scale*. Educational Psychology Service, Derby.

Lowe, M. and Costello, A. (1977) *Symbolic Play Test*. N.F.E.R. Publishing Co., Windsor.

McKay, G.F. and Dunn, W.R. (1981) *Early Communication Skills*. A set of curriculum materials produced by the Department of Education, University of Glasgow.

Miller, J.F. (1981) *Assessing Language Production in Children: Experimental Procedures*. University Park Press, Baltimore, and Edward Arnold, London.

Muller, D.J., Munro, S. and Code, C. (1981) *Language Assessment for Remediation*. Croom Helm, London.

Nolan, M. and Tucker, I.G. (1981) *The Hearing Impaired Child and his Family*. Human Horizons Series, Souvenir Press, London.

Pumfrey, P.D. (1976) *Reading: Tests and Assessment Techniques*. Hodder & Stoughton, London.

Reynell, J. (1977) *The Reynell Developmental Language Scales*. N.F.E.R. Publishing Co., Windsor.

Sheridan, M.D. (1973) *Children's Developmental Progress. From Birth to Five Years: The Stycar Sequences*. N.F.E.R. Publishing Co., Windsor.

Sheridan, M.D. (1977) *Spontaneous Play in Early Childhood: From Birth to Six Years*. N.F.E.R. Publishing Co., Windsor.

Warner, J. (1981) *Helping the Handicapped Child with Early Feeding: A Check List and Manual for Parents and Professionals*. P.T.M., Winslow.

Winitz, H. (1975) *From Syllable to Conversation*. University Park Press, Baltimore.

Wright, A. (1976) *Visual Materials for the Language Teacher*. Longman, London.

Ryan, H.F., Nur, A. and S—— X. (1981) Geophysics 46,

Smithwick, D. (1975) Reading, Writing and ... in ...
Blackie & Son, Glasgow, London.

Roswell, J. (1977) The Bay of ... Education ... University
..., ... T. H., ... Cambridge Co., ...

Steidtman, M.D. (1975) Cluster is the History and Process of
..., To English, ... New York, Cluster Science, J.N.H., H.F.,
... Co., W.E.,

Sheats, H.F., M.D. (1977) Information ... Proof, in B.F.J. (1968),
..., Biology, S.S. Veraison, F.R.S., Cambridge, ...

Roswell, A. (1954) Relationships and new techniques, Cloud, W.E.,
... Bolton, ... A. Check City and Adult Education for Parents and
... ..., J.E., J.N. Wesley,

Whitehead, L.J., ..., ... in ... to ... Comments, University
York Press, Baltimore,

W.E.P., A. (1978) World of the earth for the background ...
... ..., L. S....